Is Dentistry Your Destiny?

By: Andrew J. Leland, D.D.S., M.S.D.

For everyone who is striving to get more out of life but hasn't been able to put their finger on exactly what it is they want. Don't quit searching. If you refuse to give up, your dreams will soon become clear and with effort, they'll become your reality.

To my wife Margot, who played an integral role in helping me discover my passion and encouraged me to act on it. You believed in me and never doubted the level of achievement I could reach. I cannot thank you enough for all you've done – I love you!

For my sons, Gavin, Weston and Mason – I hope you're able to identify what it is you truly want in life and abandon fear and doubt in pursuit of your dreams. I love you guys more than the whole world!

Table of Contents

Introduction 1
   Why Did I Write This Book And Who Should Read It? 1
   Who Am I And How Did I Get To Where I Am Now? 3
Section 1: Is Dentistry The Right Career For You? 9
   The Flaw In The Mindset Of Many Pre-Dental Students 9
   Ideal Career Attribute List (Ical) 10
   Key Characteristics Of Dentistry 15
      Working With Your Hands 15
      Problem Solving 16
      Interacting With People 17
      Pace Of Work 19
      Teamwork 21
      Entrepreneurial 23
      You Will Be An Expert 24
Section 2: Dental School 27
   Applying To Dental School 30
      Associated American Dental Schools Application Service (Aadsas) 30
      Dental Admission Test (Dat) 32
      My Experience With Applications And Interviews 36
   First Year 44
   Second Year 53
   Third Year 57
      Attending Interviews 67
   Fourth Year 69
Finances Of Dental School 76
   Challenges With Finances 83

- Acquiring Necessary Money..84
- The Snowball Effect...86
- Loan Types..88
- Learn From My Mistakes..91
- The Ultimate Mental Hurdle With Debt..........................94
- Closing Remarks On Finances 96

Insights About Dental School 98
- Four Years Is A Long Time...98
- Other People In Dental School.......................................101
  - Each Class Has A Variety Of Personalities...................101

Section 3: My Recommendations 103
- The Loaded Gun Approach..103
  - Loading The Gun 103
  - Raising The Gun..104
  - Aiming The Gun..109
  - Firing The Gun 111

Closing Remarks...113

Appendices 117
- Appendix A: Dental Specialties......................................117
- Appendix B: D.D.S. Vs. D.M.D., What's The Difference?125
- Appendix C: Are Dentists Really Doctors?...................126
- Appendix D: Useful Links And Contact Information.....128
  - Useful Links: 128
  - Contact Information:..129

Introduction

Why Did I Write This Book and Who Should Read It?

If you've picked up this book, it is likely that you are inclined toward a career in healthcare, are considering dentistry, but are unsure of whether it's the right path to take. Perfect. Thank you for making the decision to read my book. I'm really glad you did. I spent quite a bit of time and energy on this dilemma, myself, and now I'm on the other end. I know there are others out there who are facing this same decision, and I think it would be a shame to let all the knowledge and insight I've gained go to waste. I am a big proponent of the dissemination of useful knowledge, so people don't have to "reinvent the wheel" more often than is necessary. It's true that each person is different, and what is a good path for one person may not be right for another. My overall goal in writing this book is to provide you with information that will help you determine if dentistry is a good fit for you. I didn't grow up knowing I wanted to be a dentist, I went through the discovery process myself, decided to pursue dentistry and have now achieved my goal. My process to learn about the profession took a great deal of work and I believe I can make yours easier. Specifically, my goals are to do the following:

- Describe the most prominent aspects of dentistry so that you can relate them to your own likes and dislikes, skills and abilities to help determine if the field is a good fit for you

- Outline the application process to dental school so you know what to expect

- Map out the progression of curriculum through the years of dental school and highlight some of the best and most challenging parts of the experience

- Shed light on the financial side of the decision to go to dental school and explain the implications of making this decision

- Give my recommendations on how to go about making your decision as to whether or not dentistry is right for you

- Provide my advice on how to successfully navigate your way into and through dental school

In the pages that follow, I attempt to provide information that will be useful to you. Oftentimes, this information comes in the form of me describing my own experiences. I took care to include stories that, although they're ones from my personal journey, demonstrate concepts or situations common to most dental students. That being said, I am just one person, and am not making the claim that your experience will be just like mine. My aim is not to provide a road map so that you know every detail of the process, but rather to share my experiences and thoughts so that you get a general sense of what it's like. This information will help you determine if dentistry is a career path you'd like to pursue.

I know you have many other demands on your time, and I genuinely appreciate the fact that you've decided to read my book. I hope that it helps you sort through your thoughts and eventually find a career, dentistry or otherwise, that you can enjoy every day for the rest of your working life.

Who Am I and How Did I Get to Where I Am Now?

My name is Andrew Leland. My patients know me as their orthodontist, Dr. Leland. My friends know me as Andrew, Drew, Andy and Ern. As of this writing, I'm 36 years old and I'm originally from Bellevue, Washington. I love golf, reading and craft beers. I just graduated from my orthodontic residency two years ago. Unlike many graduates, I most definitely have NOT always known that I wanted to be an orthodontist. My journey to find the career I love took a lot of introspection, observation, trial and error, acting outside of my comfort zone and of course, a lot of hard work. Let me tell you how I got to where I am today.

As I mentioned, I grew up in Bellevue, Washington, a suburb of Seattle. As a kid, I loved playing sports, and always got good grades in school. I was a good kid. The kind of kid that follows the rules, does what adults tell him to do, and generally gives everything he does a good effort. I was always a left-brained kind of guy – did well in math and science classes, which eventually propelled me into the Mechanical Engineering program at Santa Clara University, in northern California. Upon graduating from college, I'd identified the fact that a traditional engineering career wasn't for me and was able to secure a position in the field of Construction Management. After a few months on the job, I realized that this field was not going to work out for me long-term and also that I wanted to move back home to Washington. I decided that a career in Management Consulting would fit me well. I was fortunate to be hired at Accenture, a large, world-wide technology consulting company (you've probably seen their advertisements in airports). After a two-year stint with Accenture that took me to various places in the United States and Canada and exposed me to a variety of projects, I realized that this, too, was not my cup of tea. At this point, I was at a stalemate. As a person who had always been proactive about planning out his life, I felt lost without a clear direction. After a very brief stab at technical sales for a company who produced industrial lasers for manufacturing, I realized that I was going to need to expand my mind to find a career that fulfilled me.

As soon as I made the decision to investigate careers that were outside the realm of what I could do with my mechanical engineering degree, it was if shackles had been removed and a gust of wind filled my sails . . . anything was a possibility! I investigated the ideas of becoming a physician, a lawyer, a commercial airline pilot, an actor and a marketing person for a medical device company. As it turned out, none of these fit the bill.

Up to this point in the process, I had not been able to pinpoint what I wanted to do, but I had been able to appreciate many of the characteristics that would make a career a good fit. I realized that I loved working with my hands. I discovered that in order to feel a genuine sense of fulfillment, I would need to work directly on people, doing something that they needed or genuinely desired, but were not able to do for themselves. Also, I feel most comfortable in a small business environment and have always had a strong desire to own my own business. On top of this, I realized that I wanted to be an expert in my field. At this point in my search, it's like I had the silhouette of my ideal career projected before me, but the career itself was still hiding behind the curtain. I was confident that if I kept trying, the answer would have to present itself.

I was getting ready for work one morning. I had just gotten out of the shower, was looking into the mirror, shaving, and expressing my displeasure with work to Margot, the woman who is now my wife. "Have you ever thought about being a dentist?" she said. At that moment, my ears perked up, the proverbial gears in my head started cranking and a tuning fork went off in my loin... I could feel that it was right. I still had to convince my logical side, but my subconscious side already knew. You work directly on people and make a difference in their lives, you use tools (as dentists, we call them "instruments," not tools, but at that point I didn't know the difference), there is a large propensity to own your own business and you are most definitely an expert in your field. "That could be a really great idea!" I exclaimed to Margot. The major hang-up at that point was that I had never once in my life thought of being a dentist and I really didn't know anything about the profession. Clearly, I didn't have a natural gravitation toward dentistry, which was a bit concerning. All that being said, I saw more alignment with the characteristics of a career that would be ideal for me than I did in any other field I had examined up to that point. And luckily, I wasn't grossed out by mouths! Maybe if I learn more about it, I thought, this could be what I've been searching for!

I was off and running. I read all I could on the internet and talked to everyone I was able to get into contact with who had any connection to anything dental. I was trying my best to gain perspective on what being a dentist was really like. I liked what I saw. One piece of information that would have been useful, however, was a book that offered insight into the profession and what it took to get there. I didn't find such a book, which is why I decided to write this one.

My journey to become a dentist began by enrolling in pre-requisite classes at local community colleges and by me shadowing two very gracious dentists. I found a general practice which was walking distance from my apartment in the Fremont area of Seattle. The dentists I shadowed were business partners. They were kind enough to let me volunteer in their office a couple days a week, for a couple of hours per day, over the course of six months. They were extremely welcoming and allowed me to experience the inner-workings of a dental practice and the feeling of being there for an extended period of time. I loved the work the doctors did! It looked like fun and I wished I could be the one performing the procedures! I also saw the way their patients appreciated their work and their time. These doctors were true experts who were able to improve the lives of their patients by doing important work that the patients needed but were unable to do for themselves. After much time, effort, frustration, introspection, and ultimately experimentation, I had found the path I wanted to pursue. I had a new direction, but this time, I knew it was for real. I decided I was going to become a dentist.

Section 1: Is Dentistry the Right Career for You?

The Flaw in the Mindset of Many Pre-Dental Students

All too commonly, I find that the focus of college students, when considering dentistry, is whether or not they have high enough "stats" (GPA, DAT score, attend a highly-ranked institution) to get accepted into dental school. I understand why this is the question they're asking, but I think a critical question, in fact THE MOST CRITICAL question, has already been missed. What must be put before the former is the simple, straight-forward, no tricks question "Do you want to be a dentist?" If you have success getting in to dental school and eventually graduate, will you live a happy life as a dentist? The common conception among society is that "dentists don't work much," and that "dentists make a lot of money," so "who wouldn't want to be a dentist?" These things can be true for some, but this is a dangerous mindset because dentistry is a unique field. It's polarizing, meaning that most people either love it or hate it. I'm going to do my best to elucidate what I mean by this so that if you go into dentistry, you end up on the "love" end of the spectrum. First, let's look at why many college students skip this assessment entirely.

The process to gain admission to dental school is an arduous one, which requires years of dedication. As a high achiever, you'll probably do whatever it takes to succeed, regardless of the sacrifice. Overall, this is a good way to be, but it doesn't come without challenges. A difficulty that this approach brings is that sometimes we get so focused on having success in our endeavors that we forget to step back and assess whether or not we'll be satisfied when we arrive at our path's destination! Working synergistically with this tendency is the fact that the process necessary to make your way into dental school is so intense that you don't have brain space left for anything else. When you do have time away from the tasks that you must complete, you want to give your brain a break. The point is, the process does not promote you seriously considering whether you really even want to be a dentist! It sounds asinine, I get it. But I imagine that many people reading this who have already gone through the process are nodding their heads in agreement. So, my goal is to add the most critical element to your assessment that currently may be missing. My aim in this section is to help you determine if becoming a dentist is a good decision for you.

Ideal Career Attribute List (ICAL)

Before asking whether the choice to become a dentist is the right one, it is important to think about what makes a career choice a good one. This is a question that can't be answered universally because every person is unique, has different goals and preferences, and is happy in various types of work environments. That being said, this question *can* be answered in the context of a single individual. In this case, that individual is YOU. Deciding what you're looking for in a career is the critical first step to honest and thorough career suitability assessment. Although I can't tell you exactly what characteristics you're looking for, let me give you some food for thought to help you figure it out.

For some people, a career comprises a significant part of their self-identity. For others, their job is a means to an end. Long hours of thoughtful work fit certain individuals well, whereas others prefer shorter hours with much less engagement. Some people thrive in a fast-paced, highly-social environment, whereas others excel in a quiet environment in front of a computer, with minimal human contact. I can't tell you which characteristics you should be looking for. What I can tell you, however, is that you spend a significant amount of your waking hours at work, which presents a great opportunity to get fully-immersed in something you love! On the contrary, however, your outlook can become bleak if you find yourself in the wrong situation. What I suggest is that you think critically about yourself, while being as honest as possible throughout the process. The worst thing you can do is talk yourself into why a certain career is "right," when that little voice in your head is telling you otherwise.

For me, a career is ideal if you are interested in it, fulfilled by it and enjoy doing your work on a daily basis. My career, in large part, gives me purpose, and without purpose, I feel lost. I've seen from experience that all aspects of my life suffer when I don't have this. For me, and probably for many of you, finding purpose through your professional pursuits is essential to living a happy life.

I think the most effective way to determine which career fits you best is to take what I call the "inside-out approach." Rather than thinking of professions and deciding if they sound good, first make a list of attributes you'd like to find in an "ideal" career, and then match your list with an actual occupation. We will refer to this list as your "Ideal Career Attribute List" (or "ICAL"). You begin this process by making a list of traits that you're hoping to find in a career, you then rank order the list so that the attribute that is most important to you appears first, and on down to the least important. Do this before thinking about any career, in particular. Once this list is assembled, think of a specific career that is of interest to you and compare its characteristics to those on your list. Repeat this process for every career that you're thinking about. This isn't meant to be a concrete formula that spits out a hard-and-fast decision, but rather a tool help you methodically evaluate each potential career option.

After significant thought and introspection, I developed my ICAL:

- Do something that I feel makes a significant positive impact on people's lives
- Work directly on people, not in front of a computer
- Work with my hands
- Be in a social environment for the majority of each day
- Be an expert in my chosen craft
- Own my own business
- Allow me to spend a considerable amount of time with my family

- Provide monetary compensation to allow me to have everything I need, lots of what I want and donate to those less fortunate
- Have a flexible schedule
- Allow me to make a significant positive impact in society, outside the boundaries of my field

I am fortunate to have found a career that I truly love. Believe me, it is 1,000 times better to go to work every day when you love what you do. Being an orthodontist checks basically every box on my list. That said, there probably isn't any career that will fit your ICAL perfectly. Note that I have "flexible schedule" on my list. As an orthodontist, you can definitely take days off, but they must be planned at least a few months in advance. If you have a day full of patients scheduled, you can't decide to take off and reschedule all of them for anything short of an emergency. The point is, no career is 100% perfect and following from that, your ICAL will probably not be totally fulfilled. That's okay. After all, it is a career you're choosing; something where you provide a product or service that is valuable to others and you receive compensation in return. The goal of the ICAL is not necessarily to find perfection, but rather to identify a career that maximizes the aspects you love and minimizes the ones you don't care for.

In my opinion, the ICAL method produces better results than starting out by thinking of actual career options first. When using the career-first method, people tend to look at a profession and see it for its positives, while being blind to the aspects which may be unfavorable. Having a list going into the process brings both positives and negatives to light, leading to a more complete and useful assessment. Please don't get me wrong, I consider myself a "glass half full" type of person, but careers must be evaluated as comprehensively as possible. When you spend 40+ hours a week at work, you WILL relish in the good, loathe the bad, and find a middle-ground for everything in-between. You are doing yourself a major disservice if you don't analyze critically and truthfully in the beginning.

As a quick note about assembling your list of attributes, don't be concerned if this list doesn't come to you immediately. Start with things you know to be true about yourself and what you're looking for, and don't be afraid add additional items or modify existing ones as you go about your search and uncover new pieces of information. The way I've presented it above makes it appear as if I decided to make a list, sat down and had my list finalized with rankings over the span of five minutes. This couldn't be farther from the truth. The list I've presented above is the culmination of years of trial-and-error and introspection. Try not to get frustrated if making your list requires a similar process, as the end result is well worth the effort it takes to create it.

In the next section, I'm going to describe several core attributes of a career in dentistry. Before reading this section, I highly suggest that you make a personal ICAL. Ideally, this ICAL would be well-developed before you move on, but if you're eager to continue reading, at least make your best, quick effort. Compare the characteristics in the following section against your ranked list to help gain clarity on whether dentistry is the right career for you.

Key Characteristics of Dentistry

Before jumping right in to what I believe to be the strongest elements of a career in dentistry that must be critically considered, I'm going to tell a story from my childhood, which demonstrates a natural inclination I had toward the first two key attributes I'll discuss.

As a kid, did you ever take materials from your yard and creatively put them together to make something you thought was awesome? I did. I had bamboo shoots growing around my house. When I was eight years old, I uprooted some of them, cut them into strategically-sized pieces, and then used twine to tie them together to emulate the weapons used by the Teenage Mutant Ninja Turtles. It sounds easy, but figuring out how to uproot the bamboo, cut, and tie it together was no easy task for my eight-year-old self! The funny part is, once the weapons were created, I hardly even used them. What I really enjoyed was the analysis and planning that went into the project, the execution of my plan and creating a final product that made me proud.

Working with Your Hands

One of the most important takeaways from the story I just told is that I've always had a natural inclination to work with my hands. Whenever there was a project that involved tools, I got a feeling of excitement. The first key element may seem far too obvious and rudimentary. I include it at the beginning, however, because despite knowing that dentists work with their hands, I feel that people often underweight this attribute. It is easy to say "yeah, I like working with my hands," but do you really? As a dentist, you make your money with your hands and you will continue to do so for your whole career. Yes, there are other ways that revenue comes into a practice like hygiene, but if you don't perform procedures as a dentist, your practice will most certainly fail. For me, this is exciting, but for others, it is undesirable. As much as this element seems obvious, I urge you to give it the heavy weighting it deserves when making your choice.

Other activities from your childhood that may show a natural excitement for working with your hands would be building model airplanes or working on cars. Is it necessary that you did any of these things when you were young in order to be happy as a dentist? Absolutely not. My intention is not to send that message. I am, however, trying to help you get a feel for the type of person who would enjoy the day-to-day as a dentist. Although these activities are by no means pre-requisites, I would be hesitant about going into dentistry if they sound absolutely horrible to you. To me, picking up a tool with the prospect of creating a solution to a problem is energizing. If you're not the same this way, it doesn't necessarily mean you won't enjoy being a dentist, but this gives you something to think about.

Problem Solving

The second element of my story about bamboo weaponry that correlates well with the practice of dentistry is problem solving. In the story, I highlighted the fact that I enjoyed the process of strategizing how to construct the weapons more than I actually liked playing with them. I've always enjoyed assessing a situation, conceptualizing a solution and then making that solution become reality. This process parallels dentistry. Each new patient is like a puzzle you must solve using information you've gained from talking to the patient as well as that which you gather during your examination. Once you have all the information you need, you work with the patient to understand his options and help him select the one that suits him best.

With this in mind, there is more than one way to skin a cat. Two dentists will solve equivalent problems in different ways because each has her own strengths and weaknesses, was trained in a specific manner and has a unique lens through which she perceives each situation. This arises from the fact that no two issues are the same, and the skill, didactic knowledge base and clinical experience of a dentist must be used synergistically to help the patient select the best course of action.

Are you energized from my description of taking complex problems, formulating and then implementing what you see to be the best solution? If so, dentistry could be a great fit because this is something you'll do every day. If you're someone who would rather implement pre-determined solutions without much analysis, I would give dentistry a second thought.

Interacting with People

Dentistry is a people business. From patients to your staff to the public, you are meeting new people and interacting with them every hour of your workday. I can't count the number of times I've heard a dentist say that he is 50% dentist, 50% psychologist (jokingly, but there's at least a little truth in every joke).

In dental school, you often hear phrases like "you need to treat patients as people, not as a set of teeth that need fixing." It is easy to get bogged down in technical thoughts about the analysis of a patient's dental issues and how you're going to go about fixing them. Fundamentally, this is good, as you have the patient's best interests in mind. You have to be careful, however, because a critical part of doing your job well is to nurture your patients' emotional side, in addition to the technical. Your job is to treat an actual person, not just comment on a series of pictures and x-rays with colleagues, as you so often do during training. As a dentist, you must be willing to lend a listening ear to all those who walk through your door. That being said, it is also important to be efficient with your time. As you might have guessed, this is much easier said than done.

Many doctors say that the most difficult part of being a practice owner is managing staff. As with patients, each staff member has her own needs, wants and way of living her life. It can be difficult to harness the beneficial qualities within each staff member while trying to keep the less advantageous ones at bay. The toughest part is that this is an ongoing battle. Just because people are happy and the ship is sailing in the right direction one day does not mean that there isn't a rough patch ahead.

If you enjoy social interactions and are good at adapting the way you interact to promote a successful exchange with your audience, you will love this aspect of dentistry. From patients to colleagues to staff members, you interact with a multitude of people on a daily basis. Pay special attention to this aspect of dentistry when you're evaluating it as a career option. I say this because

I've heard on more than one occasion dentists say things like "If you could just remove the teeth from the patient so that you wouldn't have to talk to them, dentistry would be perfect." Getting into dental school requires intelligence and a commitment to academic excellence. Once you get out into practice, it requires solid interpersonal skills. You don't have to be a "social butterfly" to be a good dentist, but if interpersonal interaction is something that you loathe or gives you anxiety, you may want to improve your skills, change your mindset, or consider another career option.

Pace of Work

A discovery that I've made through the career evaluation process is this: when evaluating a career, we focus on the high-level summary of the job, which isn't necessarily an accurate indication of whether the career really *is* a good fit. The high-level summary of a certain career may sound interesting, but for a career to fit with someone's personality, the day-to-day operations and workflow must align with the type of environment in which that individual thrives.

When explaining my journey, I mentioned that I looked into becoming a lawyer; specifically, a patent attorney. A patent attorney is someone who examines inventions, determines their innovations and files for patents to protect these original ideas. To me, a description like this is enticing. When I dug deeper, however, I learned that the day-to-day pace of work was very slow with lots of reading and writing of highly technical, detailed material. Each day would include very little social interaction and each week would require long hours of work. This side of the job sounded very similar to what I was trying to escape from.

This example shows how the high-level description of something can sound like a career would be excellent, but the day-to-day activities say otherwise. I think that pace of work varies widely from profession to profession, makes a huge impact on a person's enjoyment level at work, but is rarely given adequate consideration.

Many skilled professions have what I consider to be slow paces of work. Engineering, patent law and technology consulting are three examples of careers, which involve long-term projects that take months or even years to complete. Significant time is spent on single detail of a project, and when this is complete, another detail is embarked upon. This is almost the exact opposite of dentistry. Nobody can keep their mouth open for more than a couple hours in a row (and that's even a stretch! (pun intended)), so there's basically no way that individual projects could be anywhere near the magnitude of what an engineer or patent lawyer does on a regular basis. In a busy dental office, there are often multiple patients in chairs at the same time, ready to be worked on. As soon as the doctor finishes with one, his time is scheduled tightly, and he is on to the next. Up, down, up, down, phone call, consultation, exam room, talk to a sales rep ... this is what a day is like for a dentist. No doubt, it can be exhausting, but if you're geared for that type of environment, it's energizing!

Which style fits you best? Long-term projects that you work on for extended periods of time, or lots of short projects, where you constantly jump from one to the next? Neither answer is universally right or wrong. The question is, what fits you best? If you're going to be happy as a dentist, you will most likely have a tendency toward the latter.

Teamwork

Are you a "team player?" Do you thrive when you work in teams, or do you prefer to work alone? As a dentist, you are most definitely part of a team, but you are the clear leader of this team. Consider the common scenario of a dentist who owns and operates her own private practice. She is the only dentist in the practice and employs a team of two front office staff, one treatment coordinator, three assistants and two hygienists. Most likely, the doctor has received 4-8 more years of higher education than every other person in the office. The doctor is the only licensed practitioner of dentistry in the office (the hygienists are licensed to practice hygiene only) and is counted upon to run the practice both from a dental treatment standpoint, as well as from an employee management perspective. Let me be clear: I'm not in any way insinuating that because the doctor has received significantly more education than her staff, that she is better or entitled to more than any other person. What I am saying is that the doctor is the clear choice as the person who must, and will be responsible for making all treatment decisions, as well as for running the practice. To have a high level of success, the doctor must manage and interact with her team effectively, by assuming the leadership role. Let's consider an example from one of my previous careers that demonstrates a dissimilarity to the role of a dentist.

When I worked in IT consulting, I was surrounded by other professionals with different skillsets than my own, but with the same level of education and credentialing. Each of us were on several different small teams, each working on a small goal to progress the large team toward the completion of a massive project. Each project generally spanned years and utilized the talents of hundreds of individuals. This situation demonstrates a true team atmosphere. All, or at least the vast majority of team members were all at the same level, and the projects were truly collaborative in nature. Contrast this with dentistry where the doctor is the clear leader from the perspectives of both treatment and practice management. Which do you like better? As with all other aspects of a career, neither answer is right or wrong, but most dentists act as definitive leaders.

I notice somewhat of a division about this aspect of leadership, among dentists. Some, usually the most successful ones, see the fact that they are needed as a leader as a positive thing, and they have the attitude that they *get* to lead and make decisions. They are confident in their abilities and genuinely believe that they do better jobs as leaders than anyone else would. Others see leadership as a chore, taking the stance that they *have* to lead, as if it is one aspect of their job that they don't like. Anecdotally, I find the second type of doctor's practice to be less successful.

If you were put in a situation where everyone was looking at you to take control and make decisions, would you like it? Or would it make you uncomfortable and anxious? It's true that not all dentists own their own practices, and this is becoming increasingly truer with the recent growth of corporate dentistry. Even so, the dentist is always the most knowledgeable member of the team, is always counted on to make all treatment planning decisions for his patients, and always needs to take at least a reasonable amount of responsibility for the leadership of his team. Consider this when determining if dentistry is a good fit for you.

Entrepreneurial

Do you have aspirations to own your own business? I do. I have always wanted to be in charge of my own destiny, and this is how I view being a business owner. I have learned that there are many aspects of owning a dental practice that extend far beyond the boundaries of clinical dentistry. Some of these include: hiring/firing employees, creating systems for how things will be done in the office, marketing of the practice, making financial decisions regarding the practice, among many others. If you own the building and the land your practice sits on, your duties extend into the realm of real estate, which is clearly very different than doing a crown prep.

As I mentioned earlier, not all dentists are practice owners, so you don't necessarily have to be. That being said, many people, myself included, go into dentistry in part because there is such a propensity to own your own business. It is very normal for a dentist to own a practice, whereas it is much less common, for say, an engineer to own an engineering firm. With all these added responsibilities, why do people own their own practices? I believe there are multiple answers to this question. First: you have full control. Most dentists have Type-A personalities and want to do things the way they want to do them (I know I am this way!). Owning a practice, especially starting one from scratch, allows owners to have full control of every aspect of the practice. Second: As a general rule, practice ownership offers the best earning potential, in the long-term. With the cost of dental school currently at an all-time high and still rising, these thoughts must be taken into consideration. I'll outline my rationale more thoroughly in *Finances of Dental School*, but with the current financial picture in place, I hesitate to encourage you to go into dentistry if you do not have aspirations to ever own a practice.

You Will Be an Expert

You will spend countless hours going to class, going to lab, studying, practicing and working on patients, among other things. What is the upshot of all of this besides getting a degree and being able to get a job (or own a practice)? You will be an expert in your field. In my opinion, being an expert comes from having such a wealth of knowledge and experience that you develop clinical judgement. This is the main difference between a doctor and someone who has merely studied the subject. Clinical judgement describes the ability to look at a problem unlike any you've seen before, assimilate knowledge from training and experiences and arrive at a viable solution. Basically, you've been around a subject so much that when you see a problem that's different from any you've seen before, you're still able to put together a plan and be confident that it will provide a good outcome. Through training, and increasingly as you gain additional experience, you "get the feel" of how things work. Undoubtedly this will increase with time.

There is an air of confidence you feel when you become an expert. I love being the person who people turn to for answers and direction. That said, being in this position consistently attracts pressure.

Do you enjoy being the person people come to for answers? Do you like being the one in charge? Consider this aspect when thinking about a career in dentistry.

Section 2: Dental School

In the previous sections, I've explained different aspects of a career in dentistry and hopefully given you insight into whether or not this field fits you. It's okay if you're not sure yet though . . . after all, you're not even halfway into this book!

As I mentioned originally, the questions you should be asking yourself to determine whether dentistry is for you should revolve around what you do as a dentist and whether it fits your personality. The wrong question to ask, as the first question, is "do I think I can get into dental school?" The fit of the ultimate goal is more important than whether or not the short-term path to get there is a comfortable one. But, now that we've covered all of that in the preceding sections, it is time to dive in to the actual path to becoming a dentist. It is quite an endeavor and, no doubt, the path and its implications must be understood before an informed choice can be made.

First, let's get our terminology down. "College," also known as "undergraduate studies," or "undergrad," is the 4-5 years, usually immediately following high school, where a student attends a university with the goal of attaining a Bachelor of Science (B.S.) or a Bachelor of Arts (B.A.) degree. Next comes dental school, which is "Professional School," not "Graduate School." Professional schools are the types of programs you attend to become trained, proficient, and licensure exam-ready for a specific career. Professional programs include: dental school, medical school, pharmacy school, law school, among others. In all these programs, the graduate earns a degree specific to his profession (D.D.S./D.M.D, M.D., PharmD, J.D., etc.). Graduate or "Grad School" programs are ones where a student does extended study on a focused topic, like psychology or anthropology. The goal of this focused study is generally a Master's Degree or a Ph.D.

To my knowledge, professional programs have greater amounts of pre-requisite classes than any other type of program. Generally speaking, for dental school, the following is required: one year of general biology, one year of general chemistry, one year of organic chemistry, and one year of physics. They also require core classes like English and math, but so do pretty much every other major in college so you're already taking them anyway.

An important class scheduling note: It is critical that you visit each dental school's website early in the process to view their pre-requisite classes (well before you're actually filling out your application). All the core classes are the same, but some schools have less common requirements like anatomy and physiology, biochemistry or histology, just to name a few. It is important to know that in enough advance that you have time to plan the remainder of your college coursework appropriately.

Because I studied mechanical engineering in college, having no plans to become a dentist at the time, I started off with Chem 101 and other engineering classes. I only took one quarter of chemistry, and then embarked on a year of physics, and that was all for the science classes. As you can see, there was quite a bit of work left just to make myself eligible for dental school. I had to find a way to take the following classes: 3 quarters of general biology (one full year), 2 quarters of general chemistry, 3 quarters of organic chemistry, as well as microbiology and anatomy and physiology, which were courses required by the specific schools to which I was going to apply.

So, there I was, jumping into the abyss of dental school applications, hopefully dental school itself, maybe residency, and ultimately achieving my newfound goal of being a dentist. I had done a great deal of research, shadowed dentists for 6 months, read all the books I could find and pondered everything until I was blue in the face . . . there was nothing more I could do. Still though, it was a leap of faith, and it will be for you, too.

That is one key point I want you to take away from reading this book: It is incredibly important to understand what dentistry is like, have first-hand experience seeing dentists at work and become knowledgeable about the schooling it takes to get there. Even if you do all of this, however, there is no way you'll know for sure whether it's the right choice for you until you actually go down the road. That's what makes it so tough. Don't short yourself on your research, but once you've done everything you can, don't fear taking that leap if it feels right. Without taking calculated risks throughout your life, you will not experience great success. The best bet you can make is a bet on yourself. If you don't feel the confidence to lay your cards on the table and believe that you will conquer the challenge in front of you, success in the future will be almost impossible. Nobody can take charge of your life other than you. If you want something badly enough, commit to success and get the job done. Don't talk about it; just do it.

Filled with a fiery confidence and an insatiable desire to live the life I'd dreamed of, I quit my job enrolled in community college classes and took the first step toward my future.

Community college went well and it was an overall good experience. I was able to enroll in the classes I needed, the schedule was reasonable and the price was right. Now, on to dental school applications.

Applying to Dental School

Associated American Dental Schools Application Service (AADSAS)

There is a centralized application system for dental school, called AADSAS (commonly pronounced phonetically as "add-sass"). Because there are so many different documents that make up a complete application to dental school, AADSAS offers a convenient (and mandatory) method to have all your documents uploaded into one place. College transcripts, letters of recommendation, test score documents, etc., are all uploaded there and distributed to the schools that you designate. The AADSAS application cycle begins on or around June 1st in any given year, for students who plan to matriculate (start dental school) August/September of the following year (so, you can apply as early as 14 months before you actually start dental school). AADSAS offers additional convenience, in theory, because you don't have to send the same thing to all the different places . . . except for the fact that you do. Most schools have slightly different instructions from all the other schools, and you have to go to each of their websites to determine these nuances. In addition, they want you to send them hard copies of everything that you submitted to AADSAS. So what's the point of all this, you ask? Good question. I'm at a loss.

Let's just get one thing straight: as a student trying to get into a program, you are at their beck and call, and there's nothing you can do about it. Get used to this type of scenario and at least pretend like you're kind of okay with it if you want to have any chance of successfully navigating the waters of dental school. At this point, you're trying to get into a school. Once you're in school, you're trying to successfully break into a profession . . . your time as an underling is lengthy. You don't have to like it, but life will be easier if you accept it. Schools operate independently. Although you're looking into many at one time, they are independent entities acting as such. They are not going to make it convenient for you, so expect significant logistical "red tape" at this point in the process. I know you wish the reality was more favorable, but if I sugar-coated this aspect of applying and getting through dental school, I'd be doing you a disservice.

The schools say that they have "rolling admissions," meaning that they interview and offer acceptance to students when they feel fit, not on a specific day. Under this system, the sooner you get your application in, the better, because all of the spots in the class are still open. If you apply later in the cycle, there is a strong chance that they will have filled many of the seats, and it will take a stronger application to get one of the few interview spots that they have remaining. Plus, dental schools never select any applicant who didn't come to the school for an interview, and they have a finite number of pre-planned interview days, each with a finite number of interview spots. If they fill spots for their interview days early in the process, even though the actual interview days may be months in the future, you still have no chance to get in because there's no way for them to interview you. Bottom line: earlier = better.

Dental Admission Test (DAT)

DAT stands for Dental Admission Test, which is a self-explanatory title. It's the SAT equivalent for dental school. As mentioned before, it tests your knowledge of Biology, Chemistry, and Organic Chemistry (although not Physics, even though it is a pre-requisite to apply), it has Reading Comprehension and Math sections, as well as another section called the Perceptual Ability Test or PAT. The PAT is a portion of the DAT that tests an individual's aptitude of spatial relationships. It's different than all the other sections, and word on the street is that it's the one individual item score that schools care more about than any other individual category. You receive scores in each category ranging from 1-30 in each section, and an aggregate score calculated from your individual section scores. The interesting thing is that scores are distributed on a bell curve, with 17 being the average. This means that it is a big jump to go from a 17 to an 18, a slightly smaller jump from 18 to 19, and so on. Anything above 18 is very respectable, and anything above 22 is top 2% of test-takers.

A general description of how the DAT works is that it is a timed test designed for time to be a serious issue. It's the kind of the thing where very few of the questions require extensive steps or calculations to complete, and many of the test-takers could probably solve most of the questions if given unlimited time. The limited time offered to take the test is a true hurdle though, which makes practicing for the DAT so important.

My method of DAT review involved a Kaplan DAT review book and paying for an online subscription to a site, which offered lots of practice test questions. Some people pay lots of money for DAT review courses. Because of the "scraping by, by the skin of my teeth" financial situation that I was in, a couple thousand bucks for a formal DAT review course was not in the cards. For those who have the means to take the class, however, if you really think it will help you study and increase your score, do it. A higher DAT score can mean potential admission to a school when you would not have otherwise gotten in, or possibly even better yet, admission to a cheaper school when you otherwise would have gotten into one that was more expensive. The cost of the review class could save you tens or even hundreds of thousands of dollars on the back end.

Anyway, I got to work. It was pretty much 24/7 parked at the desk in the second bedroom of our apartment. It's hard to stay focused for hours on end, day in and day out. One thing that helped me were workouts. We had a gym in our apartment complex, and I'd work out every day. I am a firm proponent of mixing physical activity in with long periods that require mental focus. For me the hour invested in working out is a great break, helps me maintain my physical well-being, and it pays dividends in studying effectiveness. I come back from a workout feeling great and able to focus intensely afterward. When you're studying all the time, your mind is chaotic. When you exert yourself physically, your mind is calm. After my mind got this much-needed break, it came back full-steam and I probably learned in one hour after the workout what it would have taken me two or three hours to learn had I kept myself parked in front of the desk. More enjoyable and more lucrative from a knowledge acquisition perspective. I continued to employ this method throughout dental school and residency.

The night before the DAT I went to bed at a time, which allowed me 8 hours of sleep. My mind was buzzing so fast that I got 4 hours of sleep, maybe. I was tired, but the adrenaline was pumping and I was determined to do whatever it took to focus for the entire test and get the job done. I think it was somewhere in the neighborhood of three hours long. I remember trying to make toast that morning, and the lever wouldn't stay down and I started slamming it down out of frustration. "Geez," my wife Margot said, "take it easy!" "You're right," I said. Clearly, I was anxious about the "event of the day." About an hour before the test, I drank my self-prescribed half cup of coffee; the perfect amount to wake me up and enhance my focus but not enough to make me get the shakes.

I sat down, zoned in, and the test went by in what seemed like about 15 minutes. That's what happens when you're in the zone. They give you your score immediately, as soon as you hit submit on the last question. Academic Average: 20. This was good, not great, but serviceable, I thought. A score of 20 corresponded to roughly the 85th percentile of everyone who took the test in 2009. I'd done better on practice tests, and I'd also done worse. This was not my absolute best effort, and my score was not going to open the doors to dental schools across the country, but I didn't think it would close those doors either. Mission (more or less) accomplished.

An important class scheduling note concerns timing and content of the DAT: You apply roughly one year before you actually start dental school. You take the DAT before you send in your application. The DAT has major sections focused on Biology, Chemistry and Organic Chemistry. This means that when planning the timing to take each of your classes, you must plan to have finished each of these sequences prior to taking the DAT. This is especially challenging because Organic Chemistry builds on General Chemistry, so you cannot take them concurrently. The flipside of this situation is that you have an entire "gap year" to finish up classes you need to take, which are not tested on the DAT. When you're filling out dental school applications, they'll ask you which classes you have completed, and which classes you're planning on taking between the time you apply and the time you plan to start dental school. It's very normal for students to be without some requirements on their transcripts at the time of application. Great classes to take during your gap year are physics or obscure classes for specific school requirements like anatomy and physiology, biochemistry or histology.

For the bargain price of $1,600, I hit the submit button on my AADSAS application, and was filled with a feeling of accomplishment and excitement. This happened in late September.

Because things like score submissions take time to process on the testing center's end, and there's more processing time on the school's ends after they receive the materials, my application was finally marked complete as of October 15, four and a half months after the application cycle had opened. Although unfortunate, this is another example of how testing entities and dental schools operate on their own watches, not yours. At this point, I was nearly willing to lay down in traffic to get my application under review in a timely manner, but it didn't matter. It was out of my control. For all I knew, many schools had filled their interview slots and had maybe even selected many of the students to whom they would offer admission. No doubt, the first wave had come and gone. There had to be a fair number of spots left at least at some of the schools, I thought; I hoped. None of this information was available since the first day dental schools could formally offer admission to any applicants was December 1st.

My Experience with Applications and Interviews

The day after my application was submitted, I received emails from two schools. Both schools were out of state public schools, and the emails were telling me "unfortunately, applications are very competitive this year and we cannot offer you the opportunity to interview at our institution. Good luck in your future endeavors." Well . . . that didn't take long. I was down from 11 to 9 in the first 24 hours. But that was okay . . . It only takes one.

About a week later, to my delight, University of the Pacific in San Francisco called me to offer me an interview! This was spectacular!

The interview was in mid-November. I made sure my suit was clean and wrinkle free, packed up my car, and headed out for The Bay. I stayed with my friend, keeping my expenses minimal for the trip. When I showed up to the school, I was greeted with a smile, checked in by a woman with an infectiously-positive attitude, given a nametag and treated like they were happy that I was there. I didn't let this bring tears to my eyes because it would have been entirely inappropriate given the situation, but it was so nice to finally feel like my hard work had paid off and that my presence was desired.

The interview day was extremely well-organized, highly informative, and overall very enjoyable. Every minute was appropriately accounted for, lunch was provided, and although all the interviewees were asked questions in interviews, none were made to be intimidating or manipulative in any way. The only downside of the day were the costs that were presented during the financial aid session. Although the presenter was extremely informative, effective and helpful, the amount of debt that would be incurred was hefty. This fact aside, it seemed like the people in the financial aid department were very helpful to their students to make financing possible. I walked out of UOP that day feeling like I was a foot off the ground, on cloud nine. What a great place! An excellent learning environment, amazing people, and an overall positive attitude. I loved it! Also, it was validation that the path I had been going down for the past year and a half was the right one. It all felt good.

I returned home excited about UOP, eager to start dental school, with wind in my sails about the process. My delayed application cycle was off to a great start . . . hopefully more interview invitations would roll in, I would have a bevy of choices, and my dream would become a reality.

A few weeks later, on December 1st, the first day dental schools could formally offer admittance, UOP called and informed me that I had been accepted! I was ecstatic! This was it! My goal had been achieved! I couldn't believe it! With UOP, it had all worked out so well and so easily. I was ecstatic that my path was set out in front of me. But, unfortunately, that wasn't the end of my story.

I waited a few weeks and still hadn't heard from any other schools. I was still riding high about UOP, but I was sensitive to the fact that although it was an amazing place, it was also one of the most expensive dental schools in the nation. The euphoria of being accepted was wearing off, and the reality of the debt I would incur was beginning to set in. I was happy, but a bit uneasy.

A few weeks later, I still hadn't heard from any other schools (so, 8 out of 11 were still "at large," two had rejected me immediately and one had interviewed and accepted me). I received the acceptance packet from UOP. After pages of useful and encouraging information, I reached the financial page. I remember the number like it was yesterday. Total costs for tuition and fees for the three years (UOP was, and I believe still is, the only three-year dental school in the nation): $296,000. This did not include living expenses like rent, food, car, etc. True, it was only three years of living expenses, not four like every other school, but San Francisco is one of the most expensive places you could be. When you compared total cost to attend UOP to total cost of many other schools, even taking into account the fact that UOP was only three years, it was still among the most expensive. Many argue that graduating a year earlier allows for a year of additional earnings, which significantly brings down the cost of attending UOP. I understand this argument, but I don't entirely agree with it. But, that's a discussion for another day. Bottom line: this place was expensive!

My deposit was coming due soon to hold my seat in the Class of 2013: $2,000. I was working at a retail store at the time, but that wasn't exactly a gold mine. I had the funds, however, and I cut the check. Despite my reservations about cost, I was very excited to be going to such a great institution and felt extremely fortunate to have this opportunity. That being said, my original vision included having several options at this point, from which I could choose. No big deal though. It only takes one and I had one. I was going to be a dentist!

A while later, probably in February, I received a call from Western University of Health Sciences, inviting me for an interview. This was excellent! If for no other reason, I was excited to see the inside of another dental school and compare it to what I saw at UOP. I did not foresee myself choosing Western over UOP, but I felt that I needed to see it firsthand to know for sure. The interview was interesting, but not quite harmonious with my experience at UOP. Western was a brand-new school at the time and with that in mind, I think they did a very good job. They had faculty with impressive resumes and a well-thought-out curriculum. Their clinic, however, had not been built yet, since it was 2+ years away from any student needing to use it. The interviews felt much more like pressure cookers than they did at UOP, which was honestly how I was expecting them to be at every school.

A week or so later, I got a call to let me know I was on the waitlist at Western. No problem. Very fortunate to have my acceptance to UOP in my pocket. I moved on without looking back.

10 out of 11 schools were accounted for. One acceptance to UOP, one waitlist at Western, eight rejections, and what was for sure an impending rejection from UCLA. If you asked me before I hit the submit button on my AADSAS application which school that I had the slimmest chance of getting into, that school was UCLA. I applied because it was a public, affordable school on the west coast and was touted as one of the best dental schools in the nation. Sure, my mechanical engineering degree is unique and interesting, and might add some "depth" to a dental school class, but I didn't think my DAT score of 20, although decent, was going bulldoze a path into what was an out-of-state, highly competitive public school (public schools always take far more in-state than out-of-state residents, since a significant amount of their funding comes from their state governments).

On a weekday in late March of 2009, I was sitting at my computer, when an email came through from UCLA School of Dentistry. "Here it is," I thought, "the final rejection." It didn't even affect me, because in my mind it was a foregone conclusion. It was actually kind of a relief, because the process would be officially over, and, after all, I was going to an outstanding school in UOP! It was almost April. Interviews had come and gone at all schools across the country. If you hadn't already interviewed, you had no chance. UCLA just hadn't gotten around to sending out their final rejection emails yet. Then I looked closer; the subject of the email was "Interview Invitation." "No way," I thought. They must have accidentally sent me a stock email of the wrong type. Hopeful, however, I felt a firefly ascend from the bottom of my stomach to the middle of my throat; a little jolt of lightning. I opened the email. It read something like "Dear Andrew, UCLA School of Dentistry is pleased to offer you an invitation to interview for a position in the Class of 2014. Please know that although this interview is late in the cycle, you will not be interviewing for a waitlist position, as we still have seats in the class, which have yet to be filled." I couldn't believe what I had read. I was blown away. I got an interview at UCLA! This could be the missing piece that I'd been looking for!

The facility at UCLA was much older and worn than the facilities had been at UOP and especially Western. The place had a feeling of prestige built in, like the world-class name of UCLA was hanging over the worn floors, outdated side-paneling and underground windowless dark corridors. Rather than leaving want, these characteristics demanded respect, as if the countless hours spent by the great dental minds of our time and world-renowned research had made the building this way. Like years of tireless effort and impeccable attention to detail would have no choice but to render the building weathered, as it appeared. I couldn't believe

I was actually there. Several weeks ago, I was 100% sure the interview process was done, and here I was, standing in what many consider to be the most prestigious dental school in the country. Did I actually have a shot at getting in?

We had several interviews throughout the day and, although slightly less organized than UOP, the people at UCLA were welcoming, informative, and extremely pleasant. The interviews were similar to those at UOP; one-on-one, relaxed, and the interviewers were all very encouraging. In fact, it seemed like half of what they were trying to do was educate me about the school and, at times, almost convince me to enroll there. I left the interview with a great feeling. It was a good place, no doubt an extremely challenging and demanding curriculum, but I would learn from instructors at the top of their fields. There was still a feeling of disbelief nagging inside of me – I couldn't believe this was real.

Six days after I returned home from the interview, I received a call from an unknown number with a "310" area code. "Is this it?!? Is this UCLA?" I thought to myself. "Hello, this is Andrew," I said into the phone. "Hello Andrew, this is _____ _____ from UCLA School of Dentistry Admissions Committee." "Hi, how are you?" I said with eager anticipation in my voice. My heart was racing. With excitement and joy in her voice, she said "I am pleased to let you know that the Admissions Committee has made the decision to offer you a position in the Class of 2014." I choked up. Simultaneous feelings of jubilance, confirmation, relief and gratitude flowed through my body from top to bottom. It was like a wave. I must have held silent for 5 seconds because my eyes were welling up and I knew my voice would be shaky. Normally composed, but feeling like jelly at the moment, "Really?" I said with a waiver in my voice. "Really!" she said. At this point, I pulled back the tears just enough to finish the conversation. "Thank you," I said. I knew what I needed to know. I wanted to be polite, but also wanted to get off the phone so I could crumble to the floor and celebrate this momentous occasion in the silence and comfort of my apartment. "You're welcome!" she said. "We're very excited to offer you this position and hope you accept it!" "I accept it," I said without hesitation. "Uhh . . . Great!" she said; excited, but caught a little off-guard by my immediate decision. "You will be receiving some emails in the next couple days letting you know of the next steps and there will be a deposit of $1000 that will be necessary to hold your spot in the class." "That sounds great. I'll look for the emails. Thank you, again," I said. It was all I could do to mutter the words that I did, as it seriously felt like my entire body was radiating heat from the inside out. In wasn't like an out-of-body experience though, because my mind was right there. I was keenly aware of every iota of emotion that was flowing through me. It was one of the best experiences I've ever had in my life.

I hung up the phone, fell to my knees and wept. "YES! YES! YES!" I yelled at the top of my lungs with clenched fists and eyes closed with tears streaming down. Next, my chin lowered until it touched my chest; "Thank you. Thank you. Thank you, God," I said softly. What a humbling experience. It really felt like I had been given an amazing gift. In an instant, all my decisions and hard work were validated. I was headed to Los Angeles to be part of the Class of 2014 at UCLA School of Dentistry.

First Year

Not long after you've arrived at dental school, things buckle down pretty quickly. First quarter, we had a class called Foundations, which basically refreshed you on the most important information from biology, chemistry, organic chemistry and biochemistry. And when I say "refreshed," I mean basically threw a ton of information at you at breakneck speed because "you already know this stuff." Umm, yeah, that's it . . . I already know this stuff. Turns out that community college biology and chemistry classes go into just a *liiiitle* less depth than they do at UCLA Dental School.

The way UCLA was structured when I was a student was on a Pass/No Pass system. The grade for each class was independent of all others, so, for instance, a student may receive a "P" in each course at the end of a quarter, and be good to go. The vast majority of students, if not all, passed any particular class. For those who were especially motivated (so . . . all students at UCLA), an "Honors" grade was reserved for the people who scored in the top 5%-10% of each class. You could see it in everyone's eyes the first time the Honors grade was introduced – everybody thinking "oh yeah, that's me, I always get the highest grades." In college, that worked. In dental school, with everybody thinking the same thing, it didn't quite work out the same way. The cream would rise to the top.

For those who didn't pass a particular class, they usually just retook a test. I think you had to fail quite a few classes to get sent back to the class below. I failed a lab practical, but I never failed an actual class. Although never fun, it doesn't affect the final outcome of dental school at all. Something important to understand about dental school: it's hard to get in and once you're in, it's hard to get kicked out. First of all, I think dental schools have a vested interest in helping those who they selected to succeed. Secondly, there are a limited number of spots available in each class. If they failed someone out in their first year, that would be three-plus years of lost tuition revenue because you can't take a person who missed all of the material from first year and start them in the second year class. This is not at all a criticism of dental schools. After all, they need to make money to keep the lights on and the burs spinning. I understand. From the student's perspective, however, hard to get in, hard to get kicked out.

The exposure we got to dentistry in the first quarter of dental school was minimal. That's how dental school goes: start broad and hone in as you go. We had a didactic class called "Dental Anatomy" where we learned the characteristics of each type of tooth in the mouth, how their shapes related to their functions, and learned the subtle nuances of every curve and every point on every surface of every tooth. Does this level of detail sound enjoyable to you? It's enjoyable to me. This is the level of attention to detail is required to be a great dentist. Take this into consideration when making your decision.

Concurrently, we had a lab class where we "waxed up" teeth. This meant that we would be given the base of a tooth, but the anatomy of the crown (the white part, not the root) would be ground down and/or significantly obscured. We had a waxing instrument, basically an electric pen with a heated tip, and a container full of meltable wax. You would put the waxer tip into the cup of wax and a small ball of liquid wax would form on the waxer tip. You would then move the waxer tip to the stump of tooth, allow the hot wax to flow onto the tooth and wait for the wax to cool. You would repeat this process until the tooth shape was slightly overbuilt to that of what you needed. At this point, you used a sharp, non-heated instrument to carve the wax into the perfect shape. Again, sounds easy enough right? You guessed it ... wrong! It is an extreme challenge to get the perfect contours, exact heights and perfect smoothness. You may be thinking to yourself, "Why is it hard? Can't it be done if you just spend enough time on it?" Kind of yes, but mostly no. Think of it this way: the people who are grading you are seasoned dentists who learned all this stuff years ago and have been refining their crafts for a long time; some for 30+ years. Also, they are instructors at a dental school. Dental schools don't pay much, if anything. That means that they're giving up time that could be spent in their practices, with their families, or doing their favorite activity so they can teach dental students. Because of their commitment to the profession, these doctors are generally critical, harsh graders. Some are "mean," but most are extremely nice people and want to do their part in producing the next generation of great dentists. I am extremely grateful to each and every one of these doctors, because if they were not there, my classmates and I could never have gained the level of experience and competence that we did. Oh yeah, and these expert, critical instructors are looking at your work from every angle with loupes (special dental glasses with a magnifier affixed to each lens), which lets them see every line angle of your preparation as if it was 2" in front of their eyes. They see every lump, bump, edge and rough spot. It's the best learning experience you could ask for, but it's demanding and stressful.

Anatomy was our most intense class during first quarter. We had classroom sessions a couple times a week for an hour where our instructor would blow through around 100 slides at lightning speed. "You have to prep the lecture!" he would say. I can still remember it like it was yesterday. His idea was to minimize class time because the real work needed to be done both before and after a lecture was given. Twice a week, we went to the lab to study cadavers. To those who haven't worked on cadavers before, this sounds intense and possibly a bit gruesome. It is, but there is no other way to learn the structures of the head and neck that can compare. You have to take the "gross" out of it and think of it from a learning perspective. We would spend 3 hrs. at a time, with our lab group cutting, separating, "teasing" (the word used to carefully separate 2 structures so that neither is damaged) and then studying our cadaver and all its anatomical structures.

I tried my best to follow the instructor's recommendation of pre-studying for each lecture and lab session. During each lab session, the instructors of the class would randomly select a student from each lab group to have an on-the-spot quiz. So, you got to stand there while they pointed to structures on your cadaver and you had to say what they were, what they did, or answer any other question the instructors came up with. This all while your lab mates watched and listened. Stressful, to say the least. You were put on the spot, and you had the potential to be put on the spot any or every week, since the instructors looked down the list of names and picked students at random.

If you want to go to dental school, get used to this kind of treatment. You are on display quite often over the span of four years. It starts with things like Anatomy, then quickly turns into getting evaluated on your lab work, and later to your work on patients. It's a good thing that it is this way, because as a dentist, you are frequently making irreversible changes to patients' hard and soft tissues, and this must be taken seriously. Without being put under harsh scrutiny, graduates would not practice to the level that they do under the current system. It is a stressful process, pretty much day in and day out, for four years. It wears on you, it beats you down, and sometimes you wonder why you're subjecting yourself to such punishment. That's the way it goes though. You have to remember that you're training to be a doctor. It's serious and although it can be argued that modifications should be made to the process, there's really no other way to effectively get the job done.

First quarter done; all "P"s. We're off and running! A welcome start to the second quarter was the addition of clinical dental lab work to the curriculum. We started a three-class series called "Direct Restoration." This title basically means learning how to do fillings: first how to properly use the high-speed hand piece (the drill) and the array of burs (tiny drill bits) to cut out the appropriate shape in a tooth or "prepare" a tooth. After we learned how to do that, we were taught how to properly fill the tooth with various types of filling materials. We worked on a fake mouth called a "typodont," which screwed into a mannequin head in the lab, which could be laid back to simulate the positioning of a patient (get used to the word "typodont (pronounced: type-uh-dont)" it seems very foreign now but will become a household term as soon as first semester begins). First, preparations are done "benchtop," which means that you can hold the typodont in your hand and manipulate it to any angle you wish. Once somewhat proficient on the benchtop, you screwed the typodont into the mannequin head and had to operate in a position emulating the position of a real patient. It may not sound like a big difference, but in reality it was huge! On benchtop, you could turn the typodont to see each tooth from any and all angles. This isn't possible when positioned like a real patient, which therefore requires you to use your dental mirror. "Indirect vision" is the term describing you needing to drill into teeth while looking into the mirror. At first, it feels like right is left and left is right; totally awkward. With practice, however, it becomes much easier. They say that students who are used to applying makeup every day become proficient with indirect vision more quickly because they are used to working in a mirror. I don't know about makeup, but I know indirect vision is a challenge.

Besides learning to use the mirror, the preparations themselves require a very high level of precision. To do it well, it is highly technical. Measurements of depths and widths of the preparation are made down to the tenth of a millimeter (dental measurements are always in millimeters) and the angle of walls cut within a preparation are measured down to the degree. All this on something the size of a tooth! It's hard to do really good ones. Trust me. It is.

You'll notice that in the last couple of paragraphs, getting in the lab and using hand instruments was a welcomed change to the curriculum for me. I loved it. Does this sound like it would be a welcomed change for you? If it does, then you're on the right track. If you're indifferent, dentistry might be fine, but you better really think about whether or not you want to work with your hands all day. If using hand instruments sounds horrible, you probably should find another path. Plain and simple. Because that's what you do all day as a dentist or pretty much any dental specialist.

With Direct Restoration or "Direct," as it was commonly referred to, you had a classroom and lab components, just like Anatomy and Dental Waxing. Following the same form, students learned how preparations should be cut and how the finished product should look by viewing PowerPoint presentations and looking at zoomed-in pictures of teeth, explained in detail by an experienced instructor. After learning the information in the classroom, you headed to the lab to develop your skills on your typodont. Easier said than done. It takes practice. But you have to get at least reasonably proficient pretty quickly because there are lab practicals.

Lab practicals . . . Another of the myriad pressure cookers that dental school continuously presents to you. After a couple weeks of learning followed by practicing, we would have a "lab practical" where you must produce a passing product of whatever skill you're being tested on at the time. Lab practicals take place under specific, controlled conditions set by the instructor. They were 3 hours long, which meant you could usually go slowly, but just as on a real tooth, if you do something you wish you didn't do, you couldn't take it back. So, taking off a little too much tooth structure on one side of the preparation, or angling a wall of the preparation too much could be an automatic fail, and you might only be 20 minutes into the 3 hours. Many fond memories.

The last class I'll comment on that came during first year, and the series extended into second year, was Systems. Rather than holding separate classes on physiology and biochemistry, UCLA took a catch-all approach where both of these aspects were studied concurrently, within the context of one of the body's systems. By "system," I mean the circulatory system (heart, blood, veins, arteries), the respiratory system (lungs), the musculoskeletal system (muscles, bones, ligaments, tendons), the nervous systems (nerves), among others. In total, there were five quarters of Systems classes, each highlighting one or two specific systems within the body. "Why do you have to learn about all of these things that involve the whole body if you're going to be a dentist?" you might be thinking. Well, all parts of the body work together, and to be an expert on one part (the head and neck), you must have a working understanding of all other aspects and how they interact with the head and neck. Makes sense, right? It may be becoming clearer why we spend four years in dental school when "all we gotta learn about is how to do stuff to teeth."

Overall, the first year of dental school was incredibly didactically-challenging. Some of the information was relatively complex, but the real challenge comes in the volume of information that you're expected to learn. There's so much that even if you studied day and night, you still wouldn't know it all. This creates an uneasy feeling because you walk into every test in dental school, or at least I did, with the thought "I know the basics, and I'll pass if the questions don't get overly detailed. If the instructor decides to turn up the volume though, and really press us for details, my ship could sink." Again, rinse and repeat this feeling for the first two years (the didactic-heavy portion of dental school) and there ya go. This is another aspect of dental school that pushes a student to his/her intellectual and emotional limits.

For me, all "P"s, and even throw in a few "H"s here and there, and pack up your figurative bags and move over to second year. Boom, that just happened.

Before moving on to my description of second year, I'll comment on the extracurricular activities available during first year. There were elected class officers, ASDA (American Student Dental Association) representatives, a course called "Basic Dental Principles" where dental students worked to educate pre-dental students about the profession of dentistry, dental fraternities (open to all dental students, regardless of gender), multicultural clubs, a committee of people who produced the dental school paper, and I'm undoubtedly forgetting other available extracurriculars. This gives you a sample of the types of things that would be available for you to get involved with.

Second Year

Imagine a marathon; a long, drawn-out, challenging race that tests your endurance. Now imagine a marathon where you're sprinting the whole time. Doesn't make sense, right? Probably not possible? Welcome to second year of dental school. This is far and away, without question, the most difficult year at UCLA, and probably many other schools too. Why? The answer is that second year features the collision of three primary aspects of dental school; one on the way in, one on the way out, and one right smack dab in the middle. Let me elaborate. Didactically, as I've explained, first year starts out on a note that seems difficult at the time and only gets harder. Going into second year, it doesn't stop. The didactic portion ramps up with a culmination in spring quarter of second year, which is the last quarter in which you are unofficially a full-time didactic student. In addition, you become more proficient with your clinical skills as you move through first year and into second year. The lab tasks get more complex, bringing additional demands and requiring increasingly more time. Additionally, second year is when you're being introduced to patients and getting your first exposure to working in the clinic. This is great! After all, this is what you came to dental school for, and a year and a half into it, you're getting your shot. You start with cleanings, as this is one of the least-invasive, lowest-stress situations for a new practitioner. That being said, you are still using very sharp instruments in close proximity to a person's gums, and a minor mistake could mean a major consequence. Believe me, the first time you touch a patient with instruments, you're nervous. The only

53

person who may be more nervous than you is your patient, but hopefully that's not the case ☺

So, you can think of second year as a time when you've learned enough about the basics of the body and of the mouth that they can hit you hard with in-depth dental didactic courses. The same holds true for lab work – you've gotten to the point where you're proficient with a handpiece and many basic procedures, on a typodont. It's basically like you're a relatively experienced dentist who only works on fake mouths. These things are all good, and second year is the year that you build the bedrock of your foundational knowledge about dentistry. It is a monumental year after the fact, but when you're in the trenches, it is extremely exhausting. It's unlikely that such intense demands have ever been put on you at any previous point in your life. You work seemingly all day and well into the evening, have tests, quizzes and/or lab practicals almost every day and constantly feel the burden of the next challenge coming your way. You always feel like you're hanging on by a thread. It's rough.

Second year is truly one of those things that you must "get through." Try your best, however, to study the material in such a way and with such a frequency that you will retain the information. A serious mistake many students make, especially those who have never been anything other than a student, is to "cram" for tests the night before, do well on them, and then feel no consequence for forgetting everything they just "learned." They think the grade written on the transcript is all that counts and if theirs is a good one, they have nothing to worry about. Maybe that works in introductory Biology classes, but people in dental school will actually, one day, be dentists. Much of the information that you learn in class will be useful to you later if you can retain it. It takes planning and foresight to realize this at the time you're in the classes, but I highly suggest taking an approach to studying material that will facilitate retention.

If studying never-ending stacks of PowerPoint slides, burning the midnight oil in the lab and managing the anxiety and emotion that comes with learning how to treat patients isn't enough, you get to take your first boards test between your second and third years! There is not an exact time you have to take this test, as it is not affiliated with your dental school, but rather the National Board of Dental Examiners (NBDE). The reason you're motivated to take it, however, is because you have to pass this test and its little brother (which comes during fourth year) in order to take a licensing exam. You schedule it with a local testing center (also not affiliated with your school) pay what is always a heftier fee than you are expecting (I think this one was in the $400-$600 range), and study like crazy in preparation for your test day. NBDE I is a PASS/FAIL test that consists of 400 questions, is entirely multiple-choice, computer-based, and is taken in one day over a period of 6-8 hours. You head down to the testing center on the morning-of (The most appropriate appearance is unshaven, in wrinkled sweats and a baseball hat, glasses if you normally wear contacts, with a ridiculously large travel mug of coffee. This is the classic "I've been studying for 72 hours straight and have barely even had time to brush my teeth let alone take a shower" look that you will come to know and love as a dental student.), get frisked by the testing center staff to make sure you're not cheating, and jump right into a fun-filled day!

You think this test sounds boring, right? Understatement of the century. And it's tough! NBDE I basically tests you on everything you learned during the first and second years of dental school . . . in EXTREME detail! Lots of questions about which bacteria are found where, exactly what type of fibers different tissues are made of . . . molecular level stuff. Translation: brutal. I remember around question #250 having to reign myself back in because all I wanted to do is click random answers on the remaining 150 questions so I could leave the dungeon and feel warm rays of sunshine once again come in contact with my face. You have to snap yourself out of it, focus, and do your best on the rest of the exam. After all, you don't want to have to take it again! Pretty much everybody walks out of this test thinking they failed. When the scores come in, pretty much everybody passes. If you pass, they don't even tell you your score, just "PASS." This test creates much anxiety and is one that messes with your head, but thankfully basically everyone emerges victorious on the other end. It's just one more item on the laundry list of delights that second year brings to the table.

No doubt, second year is taxing and will push you to your limit. With every challenge, however, comes a benefit. It's tough to have that many classes, labs and patients over such a short period of time, but the positive is that you learn a ton! You feel so much more confident and competent after you go through second year than you did as little as a year prior. It's like you just got plugged into an electrical socket where dental knowledge was flowing and got charged up! When you get done with second year, there is an extreme sense of accomplishment. When you turn in the last test of finals from spring quarter of second year, you know you've just completed the majority of didactic coursework in dental school. You've gotten through a big piece of this thing that many people say that they could never do. You've climbed that mountain. You've succeeded. You've earned it and nobody can take it away from you.

Third Year

Aside from denoting the end of the seemingly endless period of your life where most of what you're doing is sitting in class, listening to lectures and taking tests, the beginning of third year signifies the point when you spend the majority of your time practicing dentistry. I remember feeling elated when I made the transition from second to third year. It's kind of like the first two years of dental school are the classroom years and the last two years are the clinic years. This isn't entirely true but it's a good general guideline. I could not have been happier than to transition into the clinic.

At UCLA, all dental students were on a team consisting of three students: one each from the second, third and fourth year classes. This way, the younger students could learn from the older ones and the patients would have at least some level of continuity of care, since each team had a group of patients to whom they provided services. Each team had a home cubicle where the third and fourth year students could store their equipment and supplies. The second year student, because they were in clinic so infrequently, didn't get storage space in the cubicle and therefore needed to store their things in their locker on another floor. This meant that every time they were preparing to see a patient, they were required to "schlep" (technical term) everything they needed from their locker down to the clinic. A pain, for sure, but you were so excited to finally be seeing patients, and the procedures you did generally didn't require all that much equipment from your locker, so it worked out fine.

Let's talk for a minute about the cubicle assignment system we used at UCLA. At our school, we had two dental student clinic floors; the second and third floors of the building. On the second floor, where my home cube was located, the orthodontic residency took up a significant part of the floor (merely a coincidence that it happened to be orthodontics), making the second floor dental student clinic area smaller than that of the third floor. I'm going to estimate that the second floor had somewhere around 50 operatory cubicles and the third floor had more like 75. So, somewhere around 125 operatories serving the needs of 200 total third and fourth year students (100 per class). So, everybody couldn't be in clinic at the same time. But they didn't need to be. Many fourth year students are at off-site rotations, or even rotations in graduate clinics at UCLA. On top of that, students weren't able to book patients during every clinic session, due to patient schedules.

Although the total amount of operatories was generally not an issue, securing an operatory with assignment of your desired instructor was often a major hurdle. The way it worked was clinical instructors were assigned to students in certain areas, doing specific kinds of procedures. For example, if you were doing a filling you would be overseen by the restorative instructor assigned to your clinic section. If you were making dentures for a patient, you would be under the supervision of the prosthodontist covering your section. If you were doing a root canal, you had to book a chair in the endodontic clinic, where you would be overseen by an endodontic faculty member. Each of these instructors had a limit to the number of students they could oversee at any given time. Coordinating your schedule, your patient's schedule and your desired instructor's schedule was often a significant challenge.

So, you had a home cubicle where you could lock up all your stuff. When you could do a procedure in that cube, life was generally good. But because of the complex situation of instructors covering specific areas at certain times, you often got booked in an operatory other than your home cube. This was especially true as a third year, because fourth year students got priority (and rightfully so). In addition, after one or two unfortunate experiences, which may have included redoing work, running back and forth like a madman (or madwoman) for three hours, or getting berated in front of the patient, students figure out the instructors with whom they most like to work and attempt to book with them. If the instructor was upstairs, although inconvenient because you'd have to haul your equipment and supplies with you, that was a small price to pay for a productive and enjoyable clinical experience.

Each dental student was assigned to a "Group Practice." Each Group Practice had a "Group Practice Director," or "GPD;" an experienced dentist who assisted students with and approved all treatment plans for all patients being treated by students within their Group Practice. In addition to the GPD, each Group Practice had a "Group Practice Administrator," or "GPA." GPAs handled all the scheduling and patient assignments for student dentists in their practice. To be clear, GPDs are doctors, GPAs are supporting staff. It was the GPA's job to make sure that the appropriate students were booked in the right places with the proper instructors at the correct times. Translation: scheduling nightmare. Those GPAs, although sometimes a bit chippy, should have gotten way more credit than they did. I'm sure it's not an easy task to deal with 50+ student dentists who act as if their future hangs in the balance at every moment of every day.

So, how do you get all the supplies you need at the beginning of each patient procedure? The answer: Central Services. Central Services is basically a booth located in the middle of the clinic on floors two and three. Before each procedure, you go to "Central," stand in line and check out all the instruments and supplies that you need to do the procedure you're about to do. This is all fine and good, but sometimes there are like 15 different things you need. What happens if you forget one thing? Go back to Central, stand in line again and get it. What happens if you get into a tooth and the interior is not as you thought it was based on the assessment of the x-ray, causing you to change the procedure you were planning on doing (a common occurrence in dentistry that cannot be prevented)? Back to Central, in line, checking stuff out. Oh yeah, you go to Central all the time. What happens at the end of your procedure? Pack everything back up and take it back to Central to check it back in. Containers that hold 15-20 instruments must be organized perfectly, based on pictures taped on the wall of the "proper cassette configuration." Depending on the employee checking your equipment in, they would often look at your cassette, tell you it was out of order, hand it back and send you to the back of the line. Sometimes clean-up and note sign-off after a patient procedure would take 45-60 minutes when all was said and done. Another example of how dental students are responsible for pretty much every aspect of everything. I'm not telling you this to rant, but rather so that you understand how dental school really is. I've described the format and process at UCLA, but I'm sure every school has got something similar. I probably sound like a broken record, but my purpose of this book is to remove that coat of wool covering your eyes, so that you have a clearer picture of what goes on. Dental school, if you choose to go down the path, is an enriching, challenging, trying and transforming part of your life. I hope that you're beginning to see some of the reasons this is true.

As a quick side note, clinical operatories and lab benches are the reason that it's hard for dental schools to increase their class sizes. They could fit more people in a lecture hall, no problem. But for each additional student, you essentially need one additional operatory equipped with a dental chair plumbed for air/water and a couple hand pieces. On top of this, if you add enough additional students, you'll need commensurately more administrative staff, desks at which they can work, and yada yada yada. I bring this up because there were times when I was thinking to myself "dental school is so hard to get into, and the schools need to make more money, why don't they just increase their class sizes?" Well, that's why.

Another thing to note about dental school is that it is full of signatures. You have to track instructors down all the time to get their sign-off. This is often tough, and sometimes downright impossible. Some instructors only work certain days of the week. Others have office hours, but maybe their office hours are during clinic sessions when you can't make it in. At one point, I remember saying that what I did as a third or fourth year dental student was 10% dentistry and 90% administrative, meaning getting sign-offs, working through the multi-step scheduling process, getting treatment plans approved by my GPD, etc. This was an exaggeration, as you'll find yourself frustrated with logistics quite frequently during the third and fourth years of dental school, but there was more than a shred of truth to my comment.

I'll offer this story with regard to signatures. Okay, so making dentures at our school was about a 10-step process. That means 10 appointments. That's right, One-Zero. At many of these points, you had to go to the prosthodontist's office hours to talk about the case outside of clinic time and obtain a signature. The instructor I needed to see had office hours once per week, for three hours. They began at 9 AM and I arrived at about 8:30, as this instructor was notorious for having a line waiting outside her door. I rounded the corner and . . . 12 deep already. Sweet deal. Lucky number 13; not exactly where I thought I'd land showing up 30 minutes early to a three-hour session. "Oh well," I thought, "I have to get this signature. I'll wait." So, I waited. And waited. And waited. Probably about two hours went by, sitting on the floor in the hall, waiting to be seen by my instructor. At this point, there were still six students in front of me. The instructor had only seen six students in two hours! I didn't know if I'd actually get called before noon, when the three-hour window would close, but surely the instructor would stay to see everyone who'd been waiting in line for 3+ hours, right? When the clock struck about 11:45, the instructor poked her head out in the hall for the first time during the entire period and when she saw us sitting against the wall (I was second in line at this point) got a look on her face like "why are there so many of you guys here?" She said she could take one more student and the rest of us needed to email her to set up a time to come in. Umm ... really? Yeah, really. And there was nothing we could do. This is an extreme example, but this is not unheard of in dental school. I'll say again that it's a challenging time in your life. You don't have any control.

Why is dental school such a logistical nightmare? Why do these mundane tasks take up such a large part of a dental student's day? Let's break it down. I believe this to be a multifactorial problem where much of the challenge is simply due to circumstances. Let me explain. As a third year dental student, you're somewhat comfortable with simple procedures, and begin to learn and perform more complex procedures towards the end of the year. You must get an instructor sign-off before each procedure, have to have them check at certain points during the procedure, and obtain a completion sign-off at the end. This can be cumbersome when the instructor has a list of four students to check before you, so you and your patient end up waiting. You get to know your patients well in dental school . . . *really* well. There will be times when you're sitting there for an hour, just you and the patient, waiting until the instructor is free to come over and take a look. If you haven't mastered the art of small talk prior to dental school, you will become a samurai ninja of small talk by the end.

It's not fun waiting for the instructor, but during much of third year, you're not totally confident in your skills. Rather than being frustrated when you have to wait, you're more grateful that there is someone there to help you take your 6/10 procedure and turn it into a 9/10 or 10/10. It makes sense why you must get checked off at each point because you are not a licensed dentist, but you are practicing dentistry. During this learning period, there is no reasonable way to have you operate autonomously. Although you generally know what you're doing, you don't have enough experience to ensure that you're practicing at a high level. Combine this with the fact that you're a healthcare provider and you're working on real people. In any type of healthcare, it is unethical to provide a patient with sub-standard care simply because the provider "is learning." If we were designing a car engine or an innovative scientific experiment, there is no harm in just "trying your best" and seeing what happens. If your design fails, do it over and make some changes. No harm done. With healthcare, if you mess up, there is harm done. It is this logistical conundrum where providers in training, without licenses, have to learn under someone with a license, that makes things inconvenient and frustrating. I guess you could try to recruit more clinical professors, which takes time and resources, but like I said before, I think this issue rests more on the characteristics of the situation than dental schools being inefficient or poorly organized.

    Okay, let's talk more about the "auxiliary aspects" that come into play during the latter half of dental school. Do you want to specialize? I did. And lots of UCLA students do. Specialization means that you go to an additional educational program after dental school to narrow and deepen your focus of expertise. When you come out of your specialty program, you'll limit your practice to that specialty only. Dental specialties include: pediatric dentistry, periodontics, endodontics, prosthodontics, oral and maxillofacial surgery, dental radiology, oral pathology, dental anesthesiology (not actually a recognized specialty, but there are residencies based around it), dental public health and, saving the best for last, orthodontics. I'll go into detail about each of these specialties in the appendix. Most people who go into specialty programs start their program roughly one month after they graduate from dental school. This means that they graduate, often move to a different part of the country and start their program soon after. The thought of getting your applications together really begins in the middle of third year, applications are generally submitted in the July/August timeframe, and interviews take place usually in the September/October timeframe. At least this is how it goes for orthodontics. The other specialties vary in their exact timing and how the process works, but this framework gives you a general idea of how all specialty program application and interview timelines are laid out.

Most programs participate in the "MATCH" process, whereby a candidate interviews at all the programs where she gets invited and chooses to be present for the interviews. Next, the interviewee creates a "rank list" online, whereby she rates the programs she would like to attend in order of desire, "1" being the most desirable, and the last on the list being the least. Each specialty program creates a similar list, ranking the candidates that it interviewed. All these lists are amalgamated and entered into a computer system where "matching theory," a Nobel Prize-winning algorithm, is employed to return the best matches between applicants and programs. On a pre-determined day at a specific time, everyone participating in the MATCH receives an email that essentially holds the fate of their life. Okay, that's dramatic. Seriously though, you open an email that tells you first if you matched, and second, where you matched. That's it. That's how it goes. Dreams are realized or crushed over a few clicks of the mouse.

One particularly "special" aspect of applying to orthodontic programs is that we "get" to take the GRE. Yes, *that* GRE; the standardized test on math and English. Makes sense, right? I mean, how would you possibly bond braces and bend wire if you can't demonstrate the proper use of alliteration or solve a complex algebraic equation, right? You may be asking yourself: "Isn't that the same test that people trying to get into a Ph.D. program in English have to take?" Yes. "Why does it matter if you're going to be an orthodontist?" I don't know. I've heard that the program directors want to ensure that you'll be able to write a decent thesis for your Master's project, but, c'mon, really?!? As with anything on a prospective orthodontist's application, your GRE score must be, at minimum, pretty good. Even though the GRE doesn't directly apply to what you're trying to do, the competition is too fierce to have any mediocre marks on your scorecard. So yes, you yet again get to sequester yourself for nights and weekends in your second bedroom, at your desk under the dim light of the duct-taped desk lamp that you picked up for $1.00 three years ago at a garage sale, and learn new vocab words and quicker ways to reduce fractions. I did well on the GRE: Verbal Reasoning: 164, Quantitative Reasoning: 161, Analytical Writing: 5.5 . . . well enough to get accepted into the best orthodontic program in the country. That's right, I said it. We're quite prideful in Houston, and I believe we have good reason to feel this way ☺

Attending Interviews

At this point in your dental school career, along with trying to finish your clinical requirements, you're flying around the country to interviews at specialty programs (if you decided to specialize). The school knows this, and many times they claim to be supportive of students interviewing at specialty programs (which, they should be because when students from a dental school get accepted into competitive, high-quality specialty programs, it reflects quite well on the dental school), but this claim is not always fully acted upon. "Your duties at school come first," say dental school staff members. I'm not disputing the spirit of this fact, but let's take the interview schedule at University of Texas Health Science Center at Houston, Department of Orthodontics, for example. It was the program upon which my sights were set since the beginning, for a variety of reasons. UT

Houston holds its interviews for the upcoming class in two sessions, which occur on back-to-back days. Let's say, September 18th and 19th, a Thursday and Friday. If you don't make it to Houston, in person, on one of these two days, you're not in the upcoming class. No exceptions.

When I received the email from UT inviting me to interview, I was on cloud nine! The next step in realizing my dream became a reality! Packing up the suit, travelling to Houston, sitting in front of the esteemed faculty of whom I would so much like to one day be a colleague . . . do you think I'm gonna cancel my interview because my scheduled patient, Mrs. Johnson, has a cleaning and an MO composite on #19 (a simple filling), a procedure that could easily be completed during the week before or after? No way! A month before the interview, my mind is already sitting in seat 7A, a mile high in the sky, complimentary bag of peanuts in hand, heading due east to Houston!

My comments and sarcasm are not meant to imply that I didn't take my patients' needs seriously or that I did not attend to them. I was never the type of person who subscribed to the mindset "I'm specializing, who cares about all this general dental stuff my patients need done." I believe I rendered a high level of care to my patients throughout dental school and never took this lightly, regardless of my plans for future endeavors. I hope you understand where I'm coming from though . . . I was excited! I wanted to be an orthodontist and the residency program I most hoped to attend had just given me the green light to head their way for an interview!

Fourth Year

By this point, you've seen quite a few patients, done a good number of procedures and are beginning to feel like a dentist. You're comfortable anesthetizing patients (giving them shots to get numb), doing simple fillings and things of this nature. You're building confidence with advanced procedures like root canals, bridges and veneers, but still need more practice. Partly due to your increased competence and mostly due to the fact that the curriculum allows for more patient time, you see lots more patients than you did as a third year student. The situation remains, however, that you are a non-licensed provider who must practice under someone else's supervision and you still need to get all the checks along the way. This is where things get extremely frustrating.

Imagine a situation where you're tasked with doing a simple filling on a healthy patient on which you have done work before. You feel entirely confident with the procedure and you're ready to go, but then have to wait 20 minutes for a start check. The instructor eventually comes by and swipes her card through the slot in the computer. Okay, now you can proceed. Was that really worth 20 minutes?!? You then get the patient anesthetized, get your rubber dam properly situated (a shield to block moisture from getting onto the prepared tooth) and get your prep done quickly. You get up, go to find your restorative instructor to obtain a check on your prep, which is a formality since you know what you're doing. You find the instructor leaning over a patient, mask and gloves on, handpiece in hand, and a third year dental student watching the instructor take the reins of his procedure, all the while sporting a deer-in-headlights look. You clearly remember the overwhelming feeling of being halfway through a procedure only to realize that you don't know how to complete the second half. You know what you're doing now though, and it is ever more frustrating that you're still required to wait. Great, there goes another 30 minutes before you get your prep checked. Back to the chair, chit chat. Maybe you even leave your patient in your dental chair, happily playing Candy Crush on her cell phone, so that you can bail out of the clinic for a minute and try to grab a signature that you've been needing to get but hadn't had a spare minute.

When your instructor finally gets the stunned third year back on track, you get a perfunctory prep check, allowing you to continue. With the multitude of demands on your time at that point in life: signatures, patients to call, finding a job for after graduation, residency applications, moving to a new city, dental licensing exams, etc., it's difficult to sit by idly as so much time is flushed down the drain. You can see how, once you're competent, you feel great about your increased level of skill, but it leaves you in a daily pattern of frustration as you essentially do not have any more autonomy than you had a year before. Again, there are probably ways to tweak this situation to make it better, but most of the frustration stems from the circumstances. The procedures, the tests and the competency exams are difficult, but adding the constant frustration, mental anguish and exhausting level of what often seems to be unnecessary is what makes dental school the ultimate mental and emotional test. It makes a little more sense now why some doctors have a chip on their shoulder after they graduate. I'm not defending it, and not saying any of us have the right to be this way, but I can see why it happens.

As a dental student, you are in control of nothing, but are held responsible for everything. For example, you are responsible for having a treatment plan for each patient, signed by your GPD before your patient comes in to receive treatment. Let's assume you just saw a new patient for an exam on Wednesday, you're planning to have the patient start their treatment on Friday, and your GPD only works Monday and Tuesday (believe it or not, a realistic scenario). What do you do? Well, you can either reschedule your patient for the following week, or you can scramble. You gotta graduate and every day counts. Sounds like scrambling is the approach de jour!

What does "scramble" mean in this context? It could mean any number of things, including but not limited to begging another GPD to sign the treatment plan for your patient, emailing your GPD to explain the situation and ask for his blessing, proceed with treatment hoping that nobody will notice your lack of signature and plan on asking for forgiveness rather than permission, or any other idea you can concoct. (Please note, I am not supporting any of these ideas, but just telling it like it is.) Every time anything like this happens, it adds significant stress to your life. These are the kinds of things that are commonplace during dental school, of which you would never be aware before you're in the situation yourself. These are the aspects of dental school that everyone tries their best to delete from their memory banks the minute after they graduate. They're not talked about, they just "are the way they are." I think awareness goes a long way, and if you can't avoid these challenges, I'm hoping it will make your life a little easier if you're able to at least anticipate them.

Okay, it's the beginning of fourth year so what time is it??? National Board testing time!!! Remember the "little brother" of the test we all took after second year . . . well here it is! Most students take NBDE II at the end of third year or beginning of fourth year.

So, if you're specializing, applications are one thing that keeps you busy throughout the beginning of fourth year. The other item of vital importance (other than graduating dental school, of course) that occupies time are licensing exams. In addition to NBDE I (taken between 2nd and 3rd years), soon-to-be dental graduates must take and pass NBDE II and a clinical licensing exam in order to practice dentistry. Everyone takes these, whether you're specializing or not, as everyone needs a dental license to practice (there are a few exceptions to this, including licensing done through GPR programs, but I would say 98% of graduating fourth year students take one licensing exam or another). The clinical exam you must take depends on the state in which you want to practice. Each test covers a list of states, usually concentrated within a geographic region. Each school offers one to two exams in its location that correspond to the licensing requirements held by states in its region. All good, right? Well yeah, unless you went to a dental school across the country from where you grew up and you plan on going back home to practice.

The general consensus among dental students, dentists, etc. is that there should be one licensing exam that applies to the entire United States, and if you pass this one exam, you should be able to practice in any state without a problem. Extending upon this, it is the general thought, and I am in this camp, that different tests exist as money-making endeavors for the companies who administer them.

My dental licensing exam (I took WREB) consisted of the following: taking three standardized tests on a computer at a testing center (done back-to-back-to-back on the same day) and performing two fillings and half a mouth of deep cleaning on patients and being graded on all of it. (For clarification, all the aforementioned tests are in addition to the NBDE parts I and II, as mentioned earlier.) No big deal, right? Actually, it's a huge headache, to say the least. Why? First, finding patients with the perfect type of cavities who need the type of cleaning that you must perform, is very difficult. Then, you must convince said patients to sit through the better part of a day and stand in numerous lines so that you can get graded. In addition, you need to pick patients who you think will show up on the exact day, at the exact time of the test. If they don't, you fail. You are not in control of the situation. That's how it works.

There is one more challenge with this situation and it comes in form of ethics. Let's say you are doing an exam on a patient several months before your licensing exam and find a "perfect lesion," meaning a cavity that needs a filling and fits all the testing criteria. Great! Well, kind of. Dental lesions, for the most part never get better and often get worse. Although three months is rarely enough time for any problem to progress to something significantly greater than it is at the time of discovery, the ethical thing to do is to treat the patient as soon as you diagnose the issue. After all, a patient's dental health should be prioritized ahead of a dental student's need to take a licensing exam, right? In theory, yes, but put yourself in a dental student's shoes: the "perfect lesion" is something that is very difficult to find, and you found one. You are hundreds of thousands of dollars in debt and are about to graduate and become marketable and profitable; the biggest hurdle left between you and achieving this goal is passing your licensing exam. Are you going to treat the patient's small cavity now so that the ideal ethical practice is fulfilled and risk leaving yourself screwed for the licensing exam? Let's be real: probably not. And in the defense of the ethical side of the dental student's decision, the patient will not be harmed in 999/1000 cases, so it's not like you're making a decision that is putting the patient in a precarious position. Because dental schools are large institutions tasked with training the future leaders in our profession, they must always take the highest ethical road. Do I disagree with this concept? No. Do I criticize any individuals for taking this stance? I do not. It's just one of those difficult conflict-of-interest aspects of being a dental student that occasionally leads to mental and emotional anguish. Important to understand before you get there.

So, preparing for your licensing exam requires several steps: screening and communicating with patients, learning a test-taking approach to maximize success (UCLA did an excellent job preparing us for this aspect) and crossing your fingers that everyone shows up. I failed one of the portions of the computer tests, but in the end, it all worked out. I've learned that although you may get dragged through the mud umpteen times on your way to reach a goal, with hard work and dedication to get a job done, things generally work out. At this point, you've been accepted into a specialty program (if you've decided to head down this path), you've passed your licensing exam and you've completed your clinical requirements. You've done it! You've successfully navigated the turbulent waters of dental school and have managed to doggy-paddle your way to safety! To graduate dental school is a truly amazing feeling of accomplishment, pride and not to be forgotten, relief; relief from knowing that you've moved on from this extremely challenging phase of your life. Way to go! You should be proud! Now you make the transition from student to provider and put what you've learned into practice. This is an extremely exciting point in your career, for which anticipation has been brewing for a long time.

Finances of Dental School

Okay, so here's the fun part. And when I say "fun part," I hope you're picking up on my sarcasm. If you're anything like me, reading the title of this section probably makes your stomach churn. I've heard that the cost of dental school is the highest of any health professional school and it is rising at a faster rate than ever before. Great. Music to your ears, right? My objective of writing this section is not to deter you from going to dental school by saying it costs too much, nor is it to go on a rant about the amount of debt I, and many other recent dental school graduates, are in. My objective for this section is to paint an accurate picture of what the financial situation looks like if you become a dental school student, whether it be good, bad or otherwise. My aim, just as with the other sections, is to provide you with accurate information, and my insight, to help with your evaluation process.

There are many costs associated with dental school. Yes, there are the obvious ones like tuition and room and board, but there are many other costs that are not advertised as significant, yet they hit your pocket book as hard, or sometimes harder, than the well-advertised costs do. The first of these comes before you take your first test or perform your first lab exercise, and even before your first dental school interview, for that matter: applications. First, there is the AADSAS application where you pay a flat fee to use the service plus an additional fee for each school to which you apply. It's easy to do; you just check a box for each school. At first, you may check quite a few boxes, until you see the dollar figure at the bottom of the page. I applied to 11 schools and I believe my AADSAS final charge was about $1,600. As soon as the schools receive your AADSAS application, for many, an immediate email request for a "secondary application" is triggered. With the secondary application, you deal directly with each school, provide a small amount of new information, but ironically, you mostly re-write, re-list and re-gurgitate much of the information that was on your AADSAS application. Why? This is a great mystery that rivals the meaning of life itself; nobody knows. Oh, and I almost forgot, you *get* to send a check. So yeah, somewhere in the neighborhood of $30-$75 more per secondary application. Not every school has a secondary, but I'd estimate about 75% of them do. So . . . let's say that's another $400 or so. Total expenditure so far checks in at $2,000. This can be a major expense when you're a full-time student trying to grind out "A's" in science classes and likely working minimally at a job that probably doesn't pay well (I worked at a gym during this time). I guess the point is, plan for the expense of applications and know that it is significant.

    Next, let's talk about the costs associated with interviewing. What's entailed in an interview? If it's local, there's very little. If it's out of state, you potentially have to buy a plane ticket, rent a car, rent a hotel room (1 night is probably sufficient), and pay for a few meals while you're there. Multiply this by 6 or 7 (if you get a good number of interviews) and you're talking about some serious coin. If you're lucky to know friends in places where you're interviewing, staying with them can be a great option to save on costs. Be careful though, because you have to be fresh for interview day. You've earned an interview at a school and you've taken the time and made the effort to make the trip out. If the friend has a decent sleeping situation to offer you, go for it. If your friend is the type to blast music until 3 AM and can only offer floorspace for you to sleep on, probably smart to pay for a hotel room.

At the interviews, it is important to dress professionally. It is important to look good and present yourself confidently, as this will definitely come through to your interviewers. If you don't currently own professional clothing, you need to buy some. This is another one of those potentially unforeseen costs that you must find a way to pay for. Understand that you are being interviewed by people who have generally been removed from financial hardship for quite some time. I'm not saying that dentists are all millionaires, but I am saying that by and large, dentists make enough to live a comfortable life. The point I'm making is that they won't understand if you show up in less than ideal clothing with the justification being that you can't afford a suit. You'll look unprofessional, somewhat silly, and will almost surely be denied. Having a professional appearance at interviews is critical.

You interview, you wait, and then you get in! Awesome! You have a period of time to accept or decline your position in the class, which varies depending on the point in the process. When I got accepted to University of the Pacific on December 1st, I was given 45 days to decide whether I was going to hold my spot with a down payment. I exhausted most of that period, and having no other offers on the table at that time, I wrote a check for $2,000 to hold my spot. The agreement was that this entire amount would be applied to your tuition once you started, but if you decided not to join the class, half of it would be forfeited and the other half refunded. Fair enough.

When UCLA gave me the nod, I think they gave me 7 days to make my decision since it was so late in the cycle. As I mentioned, I needed less than 7 seconds to make the decision, as I enthusiastically accepted while still on the phone. UCLA's deposit was $1,000 that also got applied to your first quarter's tuition.

I was in for a total of $2,000 out of pocket ($1,000 for the deposit at UCLA plus $1,000 I forfeited to UOP). This was on top of $2,000 for applications and probably only a total of about $500 for interviews (I had lots of airline miles and not a ton of interviews). Still, total cost was about $4,500 out of pocket, which is nothing to scoff at. Plan for this. Don't head down this road if you're not going be able to have access to money to satisfy the costs when things go RIGHT! The last thing you would want to do is get to the point where you were accepted into a school and you didn't have the $1,000 deposit you needed to hold your space in the class because your bank account ran dry.

It was time to take the steps to get ready to enter the Class of 2014 at UCLA. First thing was first; I needed to buy a computer. Nice, because my girlfriend (now my wife) and I had been sharing a laptop anyway and had thrown around the idea of buying a second one. Every student at UCLA was required to purchase a laptop from the Health Sciences Store on campus and we had a couple models to choose from. And you were required to purchase the full warranty. Was I annoyed? Not really, because I needed a laptop. Many of my classmates were annoyed, however, as many had to purchase a laptop that they barely even used. As it turns out, it was a regular Lenovo laptop that we used almost entirely to download and review PowerPoint slides. Yep, that's it. There's no fancy dental software. Now, for the record, let me say that I like the computer and used it for all of dental school. I wasn't unhappy with the forced purchase. Still though, there was another $1,700 I had to come up with before school started. Although nothing compared to the overall costs of dental school, all these four-figure expenses were supported by my savings and a $10/hour job at the gym. To summarize all of this: if you're paying your own way through the whole process and are not independently wealthy, dental school is extremely expensive, but is mostly paid with loans. Before you're eligible to access your loans, however, you'll need to have a considerable amount of cash on hand available to cover the "start-up costs" that I'm describing.

Before you walk in the doors of dental school, you've already filled out a FAFSA (Free Application For Student Aid). This is the form that tells the federal government about the type of school you'll be attending, your financial situation and how much money you need to borrow to pay for school and living expenses. Basically, you fill out the FAFSA, hear back from the federal government approving you for a certain amount of loans, you accept or reject their offer (you can also accept a portion of the maximum amount they offer and decline the rest), and soon after, you get your first financial aid disbursement. Disbursements at UCLA were done in four installments, one at the beginning of each quarter. So, you get your first disbursement early in your first quarter (they don't give it to you before you start because they want to make 100% sure that you're actually attending professional school before they dole out the funds).

Let's talk about orientation. First thing: dental kit. It was $12,500 for the first year kit (that's right just the *first year* kit; more on that later). And no, there's no choice to "opt out," buy used equipment, whittle your instruments out of wood, or use chopsticks and call it good. The good news is that you have access to loans now! The bad part is that you're spending this loaned money faster than you can say "denture!" But hey, what are you gonna do? As much as you don't want to shell out the government's cash earmarked with your name on it, you're so happy to be in dental school, and after all, all this equipment is going to be crucial to your success, right?

Well, some of the items in the kit are used on a daily basis and you would be amiss without them. Keyword "some." Many of the items are used throughout the course of one class and then never used again. Some of the items are used once or twice, and although you need them at that time, it would be much more appropriate to have the class buy only several of them and share, or have the school purchase some and have the students pay a rental fee. Nope, you own it. You've got yourself some pretty expensive paperweights.

It was at this point that I came to a realization: Yes, I am in dental school and yes, many people would love to be in my spot, but money is money, and people are out to make it where they can. The federal government couldn't care less that you're going to be a dentist some day and does not hesitate to create hoops for you to jump through to borrow money. In our case, from the required computer and dental kit purchases, it was clear that UCLA was trying to lock in profit from us. That said, I couldn't hold it against them because the state of California was subsidizing a large percentage of my dental education because UCLA is a public institution. The benefit I received far outweighed the extra costs that I incurred. On top of this, I got a world-class education, and as I explained earlier, it was a blessing that I was admitted to that fabulous institution being from out of state (and with good, but by no means stellar, statistics). No hard feelings. In fact, appreciation. I have sincere gratitude toward the State of California for the opportunity to be trained at their finest dental school. This experience had a dramatic impact on my life and I sincerely appreciate it.

After the dental kit extravaganza, a few days go by and then it's "loupe day." Loupes are the telescope-style glasses that dentists wear when they operate on teeth. They also give us x-ray vision and allow us to see the future! No, that's not true. But they do make a tooth look so big that it looks like it's 2" from your face. Great, right? Well, yes, because you can do better work and you can save your back (Loupes are custom-built for each student so that they're focused at the perfect distance. This allows the user to maintain proper posture while benefiting from an excellent field of view. Loupes are credited with limiting many dentists' physical ailments that are common in the later years of practice.). "Loupe day" included representatives from three leading loupe companies visiting the school, setting up tables with samples of their wide arrays of wares and custom-fitting each student for a pair of loupes. Once again (you may be noticing a trend here), we had to purchase loupes. Was this a good thing? YES! Many older dentists never learned to use loupes, have been hunching over every patient for years, and are now paying the physical price. In my opinion, learning to use loupes from day-one was an absolutely outstanding idea. I think this is the only way it should be done (and this day in age, I believe it is done this way at every dental school). Still, however, there goes another $1,750.

Challenges with Finances

The obvious challenge with finances is that dental school and everything associated with it probably costs significantly more than you've ever spent on anything and is probably far more than any salary you've ever earned. You owe a lot of money and somehow must repay all of it with plenty of interest added on top. I'm not going to dwell on the emotional weight that comes along with significant debt. This is not a Debbie Downer session. What I am going to do is highlight aspects of the process of acquiring money that you may not be familiar with, present aspects of finances that are not apparently obvious and offer my recommendation for how to wrap your mind around dental school debt without driving yourself crazy.

Acquiring Necessary Money

You think to yourself "I am working my butt off at school every day, laying down at the mercy of the instructors who have a hand in my fate, and I'm going into a ton of debt. That debt is constantly accruing interest that I'll have to pay back. They at least have to make the process of getting loans easy, right?" Well, I'm not going to say it's hard from the standpoint that dental students get denied for loans that they need, because they don't (as far as I know). But, there are far more hoops to jump through in the process than you would ever think. As has been explained, no loan person you're dealing with gives you any level of added respect for being in dental school. To them, you're a profit-making customer, just like anyone else. I don't say this as a shot at them; it is a business transaction. Fair enough. I tell you this for you; so you know going into it, which hopefully will be one less rude awakening than you'd otherwise have.

As I mentioned, you fill out a FAFSA to get loans. It's not too extensive, but the catch is, it asks for your parents' financial information. I started dental school when I was 28 years old, many years removed from being supported by my parents! Plus, they're divorced, which further complicates things. I plead my case to no avail. They said I had to enter my parents' information in order to be eligible to receive the maximum amount of loan money, be eligible for certain scholarships and be eligible for the lowest interest rates. Is this unbelievable to anyone else?!? At the age of 22 or 23 at minimum, I have to imagine that most newly-minted dental students are not being supported by their parents. My dad was not a big fan of having to provide his financial information and I can't say that I blame him. It makes no sense why he would have to do so. This is another instance where you have no bargaining power as a student. You need loan money and you must deal with the people who are giving loans. It works out in the end, but not as seamlessly as you'd guess.

The loan money comes in four installments throughout the year. You receive a lump sum at the beginning of each quarter. If you need more money than you initially accept, you can probably get it, but you must place a formal request, this request has to get processed, you accept the offer, the acceptance is processed and then eventually you receive the money. I only had to deal with this situation at one point in time, and I think it took around six weeks to get the extra money. What do you get to do in the interim while you're waiting for the money? Figure it out. That becomes a theme of all aspects of dental school: figuring it out. That's why, if you're going to go through it on your own dime, you need to plan as well as possible and wrap your mind around this idea because issues will inevitably arise.

The lump sum disbursements accounted for the standard cost of tuition and fees and projected living expenses. The lump sums did not increase for one-time costs like loupes, your dental kit (although, most people chose the payment option, which cost more in interest but enabled payments to be spread out), or the multitude of standardized tests that you "get" to take along the way (more on the financial aspect of those, shortly). So, you must budget accordingly. You can ask for more money to cover these costs, but as you do that, your interest rate can increase on additional money you take out. Let me delve into that concept in greater detail.

The Snowball Effect

When speaking about dental school loans before they're withdrawn, most people, with a crazed, fanatical look on their faces will tell you "Take out as little as you can! Live like a miser! You'll be paying your loans down for years and if you take out too much, you'll stand no chance!" These are the same people, who, after you finish dental school will say "Wow, you're a dentist. I wish I was a dentist. All dentists are rich!" The point is, they don't know what they're talking about on either count. They are making impulsive comments without having adequate information about the subject on which they're remarking. That's fine, as long as you don't take their comments to heart. It is hard to politely ignore this group, but is necessary for your sanity.

Now, please don't think for a second that I'm not advocating frugality with loan money. I most definitely am in full support of this concept. The difference between me and the masses is that I'm not going to get hysterical about it and make you feel like a horrible person because you went into hundreds of thousands of dollars of debt to pay for tuition, fees and cost of living. After all, becoming a dentist is a good thing, takes a lot of hard work and whether or not you have a family member who's willing to foot the bill is completely outside of your control.

Dental school tuition and fees aside, there is a reasonable portion of your loans that is discretionary, meaning that you decide how much to spend. I think the most important thing is to keep the larger, fixed costs under control. Try your best not to rent an expensive apartment or house. Try your best to avoid any type of a car payment and avoid owning a car that you expect will to break down and require you to pay unexpected lump sums. Don't eat out every day – plan meals, buy food from the grocery store and cook as much as you can. With all this said, you won't be perfect. In fact, you might be far from it. Dental school is hard and extremely demanding. When you're studying until midnight, you haven't eaten and you have to get up early the next morning, buy a sandwich for goodness sake! What I advise against is forming unnecessary habits that cost you money on an ongoing basis. By setting your baseline expenses relatively low and avoiding the creation of expensive habits, you can get away with having some fun here and there when you get free time, without sending your debt load through the roof. Be proud that you're in dental school. Don't let the cost of school be a sticking point for you every time you think about it or see an interest payment. I advise that you keep track of how much debt you're in at all times and own it.

The main reason I have clear advice on this issue is because I did the opposite. I took the "I don't want to see it" approach and would cringe any time the topic of loans and debt came up. I essentially felt badly the whole time I was in school because of the debt I was creating. Don't do this. It's a bad way to be. Stare the numbers in the face up front, own what they'll be and estimate how long and how much you'll have to pay at the end of it all. If it works for you, take out the loans and never look back.

In my experience, the psychological side of borrowing a massive amount of money is the most difficult part. I alluded to what I mean in the last paragraph with my comment about feeling like you're doing something bad by creating debt. Of course it's not ideal, but if you analyzed the information beforehand, decided it was a plan that worked for you, there's no reason to feel like you're doing something bad. Another mistake I made was that I basically never spent a discretionary dime . . . on anything. I brought lunch every day, I never treated myself to any superfluous purchases and often restricted myself from recreational activities with friends that cost more than $20. I wouldn't even buy a soda from a vending machine or download a song off of iTunes for $1! In general, my frugal approach was good, but I took it too far. For your mental well-being, I don't recommend following suit. My saving grace was that I had my wife, who would remind me that it's necessary to spend some money and have fun once in a while. Dental school is taxing on its own, and although you need to live like a student, that doesn't mean you shouldn't ever treat yourself. Four hard years of dental school is a long time; far too long to "just get through it." Keep the rewards somewhat small, and not overly frequent, but I advocate building in a reasonable amount of "fun money" into each financial aid disbursement.

Loan Types

The first loans you take out are Federal Direct Unsubsidized Loans. For my first two years of dental school, Federal Direct Subsidized Loans also existed, but have since been discontinued. "Subsidized" means that the loan doesn't start accruing interest until you begin repayment, which happens six months after you graduate. With unsubsidized, the loan begins accruing interest as soon as you take out the money. I'm going to give a simplified example to demonstrate the difference between the two types: Let's say you take out a $75,000 subsidized loan at 5% annual interest to cover all expenses for your first year of dental school – pretty realistic. At the time you begin repayment, the "principal" or base amount that you'll owe on this loan will be $75,000 and your accrued interest will be $0.

Now let's assume a different scenario with everything the same except the loan is "unsubsidized" instead of "subsidized." With the unsubsidized loan, interest starts accruing the day you take the money out. Remember, we assumed 5% annual interest. So, you take the loan out during your first year. As I've explained, the $75,000 gets disbursed in four lump sums, one at the beginning of each quarter. What actually happens, if they are unsubsidized, is each disbursement is treated as a separate loan, which starts accruing interest on its date of disbursement. For simplification purposes, let's assume that the entire amount of $75,000 was disbursed in the middle of year 1, leaving 3.5 years until graduation. Not a realistic scenario, but this is hypothetical, for understanding. Okay, get ready to learn how the machine builds up steam and gets cranking!

After year 1, $75,000 accrues $1,875 in interest. So, at the end of year 1, your statement will say that you owe "$75,000 in principal, $1,875 in interest, for that loan." Not too bad, right? Following year 2, you'll have "$75,000 in principal, $5,625 in interest." Following year 3, you'll have "$75,000 in principal, $9,375 in interest." Following year 4, you'll have "$75,000 in principal, $13,125 in interest." So, by the time you graduate, instead of the $75,000 you actually borrowed, you'll owe $88,125! The fact that the loan is unsubsidized increases the balance by 17.5% by the time you graduate, as compared to what a subsidized loan of the same amount would have been!

Okay, okay, so you're thinking $13,125 in interest, that's not *that* bad. But then it dawns on you that this is just for year 1. Let's assume you take out equivalent loans for years 2, 3 and 4. Assuming a consistent $75,000/year, your loan statement would look like this at graduation: "$300,000 in principal, $30,000 in interest." It doesn't take a math whiz to figure out that this is 10%. 10%?!? I thought the rate was 5%? Yeah, it is . . . 5% *per year*.

Okay, so unfortunately there are other aspects of this situation that work against you, that you need to know about. Stop, calm down, breathe . . . okay, let's continue.

When you graduate, interest "compounds," meaning that the interest you've accrued combines with your principal balance, and then that amount also begins to accrue interest. So, one minute after you begin repayment, your loan statement will look like this: "$330,000 in principal, $0 in interest." So now, interest builds at 5%/year on $330,000, instead of $300,000. This is bad for you. It depends what kind of loan you have with regard to how often it compounds. It could compound every day, week, month, year, or at some other interval. The rule is that compounding less often is better – it costs you less money. This compounding continues to take place for each dollar of the principal and interest until it is paid off.

So, we've learned about subsidized and unsubsidized loans. Subsidized is better, but they don't exist anymore. So, the first "X" amount of your loan money will be in unsubsidized loans at whatever rate the government is offering (mainly driven by the state of the economy) at the time when you take out the loan. In my experience, they'll give you a decent amount in unsubsidized loans, but you may need more. If you need more, you can apply for "Grad Plus" loans, which are also government-funded. They are always at a higher interest rate, however. I had some loans as high as 7.9%, which is ludicrous. Fortunately, I was able to pay off these extremely high interest loans within my first two years in practice. You do the math. It makes me cringe. On that happy note, I'll lead you into my next section.

Learn from My Mistakes

The first thing I did wrong was turn a blind eye to everything that was going on financially. I figured "it's going to be what it's going to be" and got a pit in my stomach every time the topic of loans came up. What I did well was that I was frugal. I thought that being aware of my financial situation was irrelevant, as long as I minimized spending. Financially, that's not incorrect. But it led to emotional turmoil! A more fruitful approach would have been to preemptively make concrete projections of what my expenses would be over my four years of dental school, estimate interest at each time point, and to frequently monitor the situation to make sure I was staying on track. The problem with my approach is that I would endure hunger pangs to save $1 on what it would have cost me to buy a granola bar.

Afterward, this would lead to feelings of resentment toward what I was doing because "I can't even afford a damn granola bar!" Unnecessary, counter-productive, and I have nobody to blame but myself. You probably think I'm a little nuts. You're probably right. Regardless, the point is, a more effective method would have been to take a proactive approach to my financial planning. If I needed to cut back to hit my desired numbers, I could do so. Choosing to rent an apartment that is $50 less than another one would have been pretty easy. If I did that, there's 50 granola bars I could have bought every month without changing the overall budget! The mental reward for taking this alternative approach would have paid huge dividends and cost me nothing! I strongly encourage you to learn from my mistakes and take a proactive approach to managing your finances.

The other major mistake I made was taking out a lot of high-interest debt early in the game. Part of it was out of my control, but I still could have done a better job. Throughout my first year, my wife and I were planning our wedding (which was not a cheap endeavor), I was paying out-of-state tuition (Which, surprisingly, was not much higher than in-state tuition, but still significant. I was able to get in-state tuition for years 2-4, however.) and we were not yet living in university housing, which made first year our most expensive housing year of our four in Los Angeles. Add the dental kit, loupes and a honeymoon on top of that and it meant I was maxing out my subsidized, unsubsidized and grad plus loans. Now, I had a lot of life events going on that made sense timewise, seeing as I started dental school when I was 28 years old. Could we have been more conservative with our spending? Yeah, we could have downsized the wedding and lived in a smaller apartment. I did, however, sell my car and replace it with a used Huffy I got for $40 off of Craigslist. I also had a school-subsidized bus pass that gave me an "out" if the Huffy got a flat tire. As you can see, it's not like we were living the "high life." Still though, taking a more active role in minimizing the amount of high-interest debt that I took out early would have been prudent in order to minimize interest. If possible, I suggest you do the same.

A word to the wise: bikes get stolen in dental school, or any school for that matter. If you plan on riding a bike, do yourself a favor and don't own one of the nicest bikes on the rack. Buy a used bike that functions well but is not impressive to look at. This way, the upfront cost is minimal, and you don't have to worry about it being stolen. The mindset of "function over fashion" pays dividends when you're trying to keep costs low.

Here's a summary of the key takeaways from this section:

- You must have a significant amount of cash on hand in order to apply and interview for dental school (for me, it was about $4,500, which does not include the $1,700 laptop or the $1,750 loupes I bought once school started, before loan money was available).
- Loans that you take out early in dental school cost more than the same amount of money you take out later in dental school.
- Interest rates get higher as you take out larger sums of money in any given year.

- Frugality is important, but it should not be taken to the extreme.
- The "healthiest" approach to dental school finances is to map out projected costs beforehand, monitor your loan balance as you progress, and don't give it a second thought as long as you're staying on track.

The Ultimate Mental Hurdle with Debt

For me, there was an interesting interplay going on throughout dental school between my success as a student and the balance in my loan portfolio. It was an inversely-proportional relationship. As a student, you are measured by your test scores, grades, ability to pass a lab practical, participation in leadership, etc. Towards the end of dental school, you are looked upon highly if you successfully gain entry into a graduate program in a competitive specialty, especially if the program you got accepted into is highly-regarded. The funny thing is, the federal government couldn't care less about your test scores, grades, service to the community or the program that you'll be starting after graduation. Your balance keeps growing . . . and growing . . . and growing. There were a few instances throughout school where I'd succeed by earning excellent grades, doing great work in the clinic and getting accepted into my orthodontic residency program. I'd be in a great mood . . . until I received an interest notice. Believe me, when you learn that it's costing you something like $44 just to wake up in the morning (weekends included), you get less happy about things really quickly. Loans have a way creeping back into your mental picture right at the times when you're kind of beginning to forget about them. They're good at that.

Again, I want to emphasize that I didn't handle the financial aspect of dental school the way that I hope you do: lay out the costs as accurately as you can beforehand, build in a "safety factor" in case costs are higher than you anticipate they should be, and then ask yourself "is four years of hard work and this much debt worth it to be a dentist?" If the answer is "yes," act like you're in debt before you really are and accept the debt as it comes. It could almost be looked at a badge of honor once you've gotten through the repayment process. When the government emails you about your debt load or daily interest accrual, it should be of no surprise because you already know. This is the "healthy" way to go about accruing dental school debt.

Dental school is expensive. For me, my total debt load upon graduating from residency was just shy of $350,000. This included about $282,000 of principal and $67,000 in interest that accrued while I was in school. The high level of interest is due me taking out lots of high-interest debt at the beginning of dental school, combined with the fact that I spent an additional two years specializing (during which, interest on unsubsidized loans was actively accruing). Dental school will almost certainly be the biggest investment you'll have made up to that point in your life. That being said, try not to let the cost scare you. Instead, empower yourself by staring the true costs in the teeth as best you can, get it all down on paper, and decide one way or the other. Don't feel pressure when making this decision. Either a "yes" or a "no" can be the right decision, depending on the person. If your answer is "no," and you go about your search to find the right fit as vigorously as you have so far by picking up this book, I'm confident you'll find your ideal career. If your answer is "yes" though, there's really no choice but to be "all in." There is really no "try" with dentistry. It's a huge commitment that will last many years, likely a lifetime. As a dentist, as long as you plan carefully, I believe that you'll be able to pay off your debt and still live a nice life. If you incur the debt and decide you don't like dentistry, however, you have most likely created a disaster. For a person in this situation, dentistry could be referred to as the "golden handcuffs." Highly lucrative, but you'll have dramatically limited your ability to make choices. If you love dentistry, you'll do great! If you don't, however, the outlook could be bleak.

Closing Remarks on Finances

Did you hate reading that section as much as I hated writing it?!? What a downer! Please, please, please, don't let the section you just read be the determining factor in whether or not you become a dentist. Dentistry is an amazing field in which you get to make significant impacts on the lives of others, you are challenged both mentally and physically, and you can earn a great living. It is an incredible profession and I am grateful every day that I was led down this path. I feel fulfilled, stimulated and enjoy my work every day. I am proud to be accomplished and call myself a doctor. I have a lot of loans, but am confident that I will be able to pay them off without significant hardship. If I could do it over again, I wouldn't do it any other way. If dentistry sounds like a great fit for you, please heed my advice given earlier in this section and DO IT! I want you to experience the high-level fulfillment, satisfaction and pride that I feel!

Insights about Dental School

Four Years is a Long Time

Dental school is intense. Oh yeah, and it's long. The length of a marathon at a sprint's pace, remember? Here's the interesting thing – not everybody in the world is a dentist, or a doctor, or something similar. Many of your friends, family members, acquaintances, etc. will not really understand what you're going through. That's okay, as it's not their job to empathize, as doing what you're doing will be completely your choice. That being said, it's hard. And it lasts a long time.

Say, for instance, you were doing something super-intense for the period of six months. Your friends rarely heard from you and when they did it was likely brief. You weren't available to participate in your regular social activities. In their minds, for this period, you were a shell of your real self. After six months went by, you could re-assimilate yourself into your old ways and, in my estimation, you could probably pick up with your friends right where you left off; a slight blip on the radar which is now over and done with. How about four years? It's kind of like, the minute you enter dental school your life outside largely goes on pause, but everyone else's does not. People continue to live, develop and progress. You are progressing at a rapid rate, but this is heavily tilted in one direction – dentistry. You are probably not enhancing relationships with people outside of dental school or buying a house or having a baby. Some people do one of these while in school, and maybe a small handful manage all of them, but these people are in the minority. Most people are "nose to the grindstone" with only the occasional break which they spend basically catching their breath before the bell dings to step back in the ring and begin the next round.

I need to be careful not to be overly dramatic. Your time is not entirely taken up by school. You have periods of opportunity to talk to friends, even hang out sometimes if they live close by, visit family occasionally, and pursue some of the hobbies that you had before school began. The challenge is that the mental demands of dental school take a toll and you're usually left feeling "brain dead" by the time the break rolls around (like after Finals, for instance). Quite often, the only thing you want to do is go on a Netflix binge for three straight days. There's no problem with this at all, but you can see how if your break time is limited and you spend it on the couch, you won't make much contact with those to whom you're close. On the contrary, you need time to relax and recharge. What's an aspiring dentist to do? What can I say, dental school is a challenging time in your life.

Even if your supporters start out enthusiastic about what you're doing, this may fade as time goes on. It's hard for someone who has not gone through dental school or something similar to be sympathetic for such a long stretch. Then, if you decide to specialize, the race you're running gets even longer! Tack on two to six more years depending on your specialty . . . when you're in it, it can seem like an eternity. And, in most cases, despite the toll that going to school for additional years may take on your relationships, you'll probably do it anyway. I did.

And I'm happy, because I absolutely love being an orthodontist. It's important to note though, that this decision comes with consequences. The point I'm trying to demonstrate is that most of your time during dental school will have to be allotted to just that; dental school. There's not enough time for everything else in your life, which can lead to some degree of regression in these areas. That's not to say these relationships and hobbies can't be revived later, but this is a concept that's good to wrap your head around before you get in the thick of everything.

A positive note about relationships is that you will probably meet people who will eventually become some of your best friends, in dental school. Actually, it is common for two people to meet in school and end up getting married! Every class has one or two couples like that. Even if it doesn't go quite this far for you, most people end up with classmates with whom they stay in close touch well after dental school ends. Dental school is a grueling, stressful time that takes a serious emotional toll on each student. The challenge brings the members of the class together. Everyone is taking the same classes, the same tests and the same lab practicals at the same time. You end up interacting with the people in your class so much that strong bonds form. With the handful of classmates with whom you mesh well, those bonds tend to grow even deeper. I made a group of amazing friends in dental school and I'm sure we'll stay in contact for the rest of our lives.

Other People in Dental School

Within each dental school class, there are people from a wide range of backgrounds. These differences come not just in education, but also work histories, places of origin, ethnicities, religious affiliations, socio-economic statuses, as well as personalities and mindsets toward dentistry. I think this diversity within each class is created by admissions committees on purpose, as it generates a dynamic learning environment for each student. In addition, it makes sense that when selecting the best overall applicants to fill the class, a reasonable amount of diversity of backgrounds is to be expected.

Each Class has a Variety of Personalities

As I've demonstrated in earlier sections, dentistry is an all-encompassing career, where it's common for the doctor to wear many hats. It is not uncommon for the same person to be the practitioner, practice owner, boss, human resources manager and marketer. With this in mind, however, nobody is good at everything. With this in mind, it makes sense that there are many different personalities within a dental school class. Some people have an artist's eye, and value exceptionally esthetic work over all else. Others see dentistry simply as caring for people's health and are more concerned with the functionality and longevity of their work, with esthetics taking a back seat. Some people adopt a more global view and see dentistry as a way to help others and enhance the world, not giving as much attention to the details. Others are very technically-minded and see dental school as an extension of the scientific research they completed during their undergraduate studies.

Some dentists are very social and place high value on connecting with their patients and forming a bond. Others are more introverted and believe that the greatest service they can provide is delivering the highest quality work. In my opinion, none of these are superior to others. The common threads are that everyone is intelligent, driven and knows how to produce results on tests, requirements and assignments. Without these qualities, someone else would have taken their spot in the class. Beyond this, however, the range of personalities is widespread, which makes for an engaging experience both within the realm of dentistry and outside it.

Section 3: My Recommendations

Dentistry is an amazing profession... for the right person. Because it is so different than most other occupations, dentistry usually either fits a person well, or doesn't fit them at all. This is one of the biggest decisions in your life and I know you're not taking it lightly.

The Loaded Gun Approach

I have a general approach that I'd like to share with you and recommend that you employ regardless of what field you embark upon, dentistry or otherwise. I call it the "Loaded Gun Approach." A loaded gun is ready to be fired at any moment. In this metaphor, the loaded gun symbolizes you being ready and eager to take advantage of opportunities that become available to you. Good opportunities are often few and far between, and in addition, are fleeting. If you're not poised to take advantage *before* the opportunity becomes available, you'll likely miss your chance.

Loading the Gun

In the first step of the Loaded Gun Approach, "Loading the Gun," your task is to gather information. You must become a self-taught expert in the dental school admissions process and how the profession works, in general. I'm not saying you need to learn *how* to be a dentist, as that's what dental school is for. What I am saying is that you need to educate yourself on what it takes to get into dental school, what it takes to be a dentist and how you can go about accomplishing both of these things. It is in your best interest to reference websites, books and podcasts to learn as much as you can. In order to embark upon the next steps in the process, you need to be able to speak intelligently on these topics.

Raising the Gun

The second step in the Loaded Gun Approach, "Raising the Gun," is to form a network of people who will be helpful in your pursuit of getting accepted into dental school. The purpose of doing this is two-fold: 1) Acquire information that is useful to you now or will be useful in the future and 2) Form positive relationships with people that are where you want to be. Information found on websites, in books and in podcasts can be useful, but information acquired directly from knowledgeable individuals is almost always better.

Forming a network is not easy and requires you to be proactive. Here are a few ideas on how to get started:

- Call dentists in your area and ask if you're able to shadow for a day, or if they're willing to give you an hour of their time to meet for lunch.
- Contact existing dental students and ask if they are willing to do the same things.
- Reach out to the admissions offices at dental schools to introduce yourself and ask if there are any opportunities for prospective students to volunteer at, or at least tour, the school.

I know that the thought of contacting people in the field and asking for their help probably seems intimidating. It's okay to feel this way, but don't let it paralyze you. Forming a network is a critical part of this process. You have to step out of your comfort zone and pave your own way. Remember that inaction is the only surefire way to guarantee failure.

Strategy and Action. Repeat.

To effectively "Raise the Gun," you must employ strategy and action, on a repeat cycle. First, strategize which actions you think will yield the best results. Next, take action to bring your ideas to life. It is very seldom that things work on the first try. When you hit a dead end, re-strategize with the new knowledge you've gained and start down another path. If you're going to be successful, you can't get in the habit of counting failures. Instead, you must believe that each is a learning opportunity that provides you critical insight, which allows you to get closer to reaching your goal.

When deciding who to contact, prioritize existing connections first. After you exhaust this list, I suggest calling young dentists in your area, specifically those who own their own practices. While you're employing this approach, work on as many potential avenues as you can, simultaneously. Don't call one person, wait for a return call . . . and when they don't call, keep waiting . . . and when they still don't call, still keep waiting . . . essentially, this is inaction. Don't convince yourself that taking this approach is the same as really taking action. Taking action means continuing to try until you find something that works. It doesn't matter if something that *should have* worked didn't work, or if something that *could have* worked didn't work. It doesn't matter if things are fair or if they're unfair. It's all irrelevant. All that matters are results... finding avenues that will help you achieve your goals. Be focused, have thick skin and never make excuses.

One issue that halts people in their tracks when taking this approach is that they "don't know who to call." A critical nuance to be aware of is that you are trying to form a network of people who will help you, but you won't know whether they'll be of any help until well after you make initial contact. What this means is, you have to take the first step before any benefit can possibly come your way. You must consistently make investments of your time and energy *before* you know whether or not your efforts will pay off. You essentially have to make it a numbers game; the more people you contact, the more likely it is that someone will be able to help you. You don't know who that "needle in the haystack" will be, but if you continually put yourself out there, you'll find it at some point.

Allow me to share some thoughts that will hopefully make it easier to initiate phone calls and emails: We've all been where you are . . . or at least most of us. We remember what's it's like. In addition, we want to support the next generation of great dentists. If you're the one being proactive and stepping out of your comfort zone as your own advocate, I believe that YOU are very possibly this person. That's not the whole story though; people love to feel important and dentists are no exception. It is flattering when a potential future dentist calls you, says a bunch of nice things, and then requests your help. You feel important! That's another reason why people will be motivated to help you. It's self-serving, but it benefits you immensely, so grab the bull by the horns and make it happen!

Here's a secret: In life, people surround themselves with (and do favors for) people they like. Plain and simple. This applies to personal relationships, sure, but business (including dentistry) as well. Of course, there's more to it than just that, but likability contributes HUGELY to how basically everything gets done. What this means to you is that if you put yourself out there, get to know people and let them get to know you, the prospect of you reaching your goals will be dramatically increased. Be honest about what you're trying to achieve and you'll be surprised at how many people will be willing to help.

Let me be clear that in no way, shape or form am I insinuating that you should be fake, manipulative or try to "use" anybody to get what you want. Not at all. Being genuine when meeting people is essential! That being said, these concepts are not mutually exclusive. You can be genuine *and* be looking for a beneficial relationship at the same time! There is nothing wrong with that. As I've mentioned, people enjoy helping others and they like to feel important. Asking a practicing dentist for help and advice is not being dishonest or conniving. It's all a part of the natural evolution of our profession. More than likely, there will be a day in the future when a prospective dentist calls your office and asks you for help.

Here's an example from my own life that clearly demonstrates how beneficial it can be to form a professional network and also how tapping into even loose connections can be invaluable: When I was in college, my goal one summer was to obtain an internship for the second half of summer, after I returned home to Seattle following a study abroad program in Spain. With the help of the on-campus Career Center and a dear friend who was a Career Counselor there, I built a resume that I knew was a winner. I applied to every engineering internship posting I could find, and even took a proactive approach to contact engineering companies to see if they had any opportunities that weren't published to the public. And I found my dream internship and sailed happily off into the sunset, right?!? Wrong! I got nothing. Nada. Zilch. Zero.

My dad knew I was looking for an internship and wanted to help. He saw his neighbor, who was an architect, mowing his lawn one day. They began to converse, and my dad mentioned that I was studying mechanical engineering and was looking for a summer internship in the area. My dad's neighbor, we'll call him Bob, seemed enthusiastic about the idea and reached out to several of his contacts at engineering companies to ask if they had summer internships available. None of them did, but one of Bob's friends, let's call him Jim, had a friend at another engineering firm who he thought may be looking for an intern. Having never met me, nor my dad, Jim graciously passed on my information because his friend passed it to him. Jim's friend, we'll call him Dave, received my information and called me to come in for an interview. In the interview, I learned that Dave was considering hiring an intern, but not fully convinced that he wanted to do so. Dave and I had a great conversation, during which I explained that I was going to Spain for the first half of summer to study abroad. By the end of the interview, Dave had offered me an internship for the second half of the summer, catering exactly to my study abroad schedule! I would get beneficial engineering experience at a wage that was way above what I would have earned if I returned to my previous job at the golf course! Amazingly, this was exactly what I was looking for!

To recap, my dad's neighbor who barely knew me, passed my resume on to his friend who didn't know me nor my dad, who passed it on to his friend who didn't know me nor my dad nor my dad's neighbor for that matter, and he offered me the exact job I wanted for the exact period of time I wanted it. This all happened when he wasn't entirely sure that he was going to hire an intern, but his motivation increased when his good friend passed my resume his way. Relationships matter. Connections matter, even if they're weak ones! People love working with and helping people they like. They also love feeling important. I didn't make the rules, I just play by them. All highly-successful people understand, embrace and leverage this concept. I suggest you do the same.

Aiming the Gun

Develop the mindset of "Yes!"

The third step of the Loaded Gun Approach, "Aiming the Gun," deals with being ready to take advantage of opportunities when you are presented with them. The first sub-part of Aiming the Gun is to develop the mindset of "yes" toward everything involving dentistry. Be ready to move your personal schedule around to take advantage of every potential opportunity that comes your way. If a dentist offers to meet with you in her office or if a dental student is willing to meet with you during his midnight study break, do everything in your power to make it happen. It is extremely important to understand your role when you're trying to break into a new field; in essence, you are the beggar and you can't be the chooser. If people are willing to help you, it is your job to conform to their schedule. Get up early, stay up late, skip a class or a workout or whatever you have to do to take advantage of each potentially beneficial opportunity. You'll be surprised how often you won't get a second chance if you let the first one go by.

Be Strategic

The second sub-part of Aiming the Gun is to logistically put yourself in a position to take advantage of opportunities. If your goal is to spend time in dental offices, but you need to work while taking your pre-requisites, try your best to get a job where you work on nights and weekends. If you work Monday-Thursday 8-5, your chance of spending time in any dental office is slim. Have a cell phone and computer that work. Nothing is more annoying than dropped calls if you're trying to help someone out. When you're approaching interview time, make sure you have a professional-looking suit that fits properly. Also, save up airline miles in advance. To the best of your ability, save money for this stage of the process. I realize that money doesn't grow on trees, especially during this period of your life, but you have to prioritize these expenses.

All of this seems completely obvious, but the key distinction is that it takes intentional focus and foresight to execute these concepts. You have to strategically plan what you'll need, evaluate that against what you have, and figure out a way to fill in the gap. All this while trying to consistently ace tests and dominate lab exercises. Good grades are essential, but I want to stress that grades alone are not enough. At this challenging stage in the game, it will be very difficult to succeed without proper planning and consistent execution.

Firing the Gun

You've gathered information, you've built a network, you're constantly being proactive, and you've put yourself in a logistical position to take advantage of a good opportunity . . . Nice work! I love this quote:

> "Luck is what happens when preparation meets opportunity."
> –Seneca

I am a firm believer that luck does not come down to pure chance. "Lucky people" are those who take the Loaded Gun Approach. They work their tails off to position themselves to take advantage of opportunities, which is when "lucky" things happen to them. If you adopt and employ the Loaded Gun Approach whole-heartedly, I'm confident you will be "lucky" too.

It is important to understand that good opportunities are almost never perfect. As I mentioned earlier, it's probably worth skipping one Chemistry class session to meet a dentist who's on a really tight schedule. It's definitely worth postponing a game of golf with a friend to fly to Minneapolis for a dental school interview. Where the rubber really meets the road is your willingness to move to wherever the best school that accepts you, is located. Hopefully, you get into your in-state school (if your state has one), it's close to home, and the choice is easy. Since the dental school admissions process is so competitive, however, you might be faced with the decision between moving far away from home or having to apply again the following year. The decision is yours and I would not pass judgement either way, but if you're 100% committed to becoming a dentist, you need to be willing to move wherever is necessary. The choices made while navigating the turbulent waters of dental school applications are personal to each individual, but realize that good opportunities are almost never perfect, and quite often don't last long. Maintain lofty goals, but be realistic and don't be afraid to take advantage of a slightly less than perfect opportunity if it is indeed a good one.

Closing Remarks

There has been a lot of information and quite a few opinions in this book. I know, it's a lot to take in. If the decision to become a dentist is weighing heavily on you, step back, take a deep breath and be confident that you will make the right decision. To help with the process, paralleling the thoughts I've included in this book, I've assembled a list of what I consider to be key questions to ask yourself when trying to decide if dentistry is the right career for you:

- Do you have a desire to provide a service to people? To help them? Will this fulfill a higher purpose for you? I believe that for anyone to truly love dentistry, this must be the bedrock upon which you build your career.

- Do you love working with your hands? As a dentist, you do this all day, every day. It's amazing how common it is for people to overlook this aspect of dentistry, later to find that they don't like working with their hands.

- Do you enjoy interacting with people? Each of your patients and staff members is a person with a story, a personality and unique likes and dislikes. To be a good dentist, you need to be receptive and caring to these attributes. It can be invigorating or exhausting, depending on your personality.

- Do you want to be in charge? As a dentist, you will either be completely in charge of everything (if you own your own practice) or at least in charge of all your dentistry (if you are an associate in a practice). Either way, if you're a dentist, you're going to be in charge of something.

- Are you interested in owning and running a practice? You don't have to be, but if you're entrepreneurial, I think this is a positive for dentistry.

- Are you the type of person that enjoys wearing many hats? Especially as a practice owner, this will be you.

- Does the financial and debt picture look acceptable to you? Don't be scared and don't be ignorant. Unfortunately though, the debt incurred from dental school is significant and must be taken seriously.

- Lastly, try to put everything rattling around in your mind aside and ask yourself "Would I be happy if I was a dentist?" Plain and simple. Sometimes we make things too complicated when it's more appropriate to step back and listen to your heart.

I hope you have gained knowledge and insight from this book and feel that your time reading it was well spent. My goal was to provide an insider's perspective into the profession to help you determine if it is a good fit for you, and I hope I have accomplished this aim. Despite the significant hurdles involved in becoming a dentist, it is most definitely attainable if you set your mind to it. Be thoughtful, be critical, but don't be scared. Paralysis by fear is the biggest killer to you reaching your goals. Selfishly, I hope that the information in this book drives you toward dentistry so that I will soon have another outstanding colleague! In reality, however, whether dentistry is for you or not, I hope that my words have provided enlightenment and inspired thought toward whatever path you choose to pursue. After all, we're all trying to find fulfillment and be happy, right? I feel very fortunate to have found this for myself and I wish the same for you. Go about your analysis with an open mind and an eagerness to act and I'm confident you'll find your path. Good luck!

Appendices

Appendix A: Dental Specialties

My aim with this book was to help you determine if becoming a dentist is the right choice for you. That being said, I mentioned several times that I went beyond general dental education and became an orthodontist. You may be thinking to yourself "why is this guy writing a book all about dental school when that wasn't even his final stop?" True, good point. But, as I mentioned in the first section, I never had even the slightest inkling that I would become a dentist until several years after college. Similarly, when I decided upon dentistry, I did not have aspirations of becoming an orthodontist. This was decided while I was in dental school. I feel that my path to decide on dentistry was by far the most significant, and also applicable to more people than my journey into orthodontics. I love dentistry, and I love ortho even more. To me, orthodontics it's an extension onto something great.

Dental school comes at you at warp speed from the moment you walk in the door. If you want to specialize, you really need to decide this by the middle of third year at the latest, in order to meet the application deadlines. The challenge with this timeline is that the point at which you need to apply comes at a time when you're only just beginning to gain exposure to the specialties. How are you supposed to know if you want to be an endodontist if you just performed your first root canal a few months ago?!? As a primer, I want to give you a brief overview of all the dental specialties, to allow your wheels to start turning. Remember, the first step to being a loaded gun is to put a bullet in the chamber.

Orthodontics: You probably had braces, right? And you probably LOVED your orthodontist!!! Okay, maybe I'm getting ahead of myself, but many people actually do say they love their orthodontist. Orthodontists are specialists in the position of the teeth, the bite and the skeletal component of the jaws. Our training is heavily focused on diagnosis and treatment planning, as the most critical part of orthodontics takes places before the braces are even placed on teeth. We work closely with oral surgeons in a variety of types of cases where the patient needs the services of both specialties. Orthodontics is the perfect specialty for people who like problem-solving, puzzles and physics. It's also great for those who enjoy interacting with lots of people, as some orthodontists see upwards of 100 patients per day! The best part about it, however, is the amazing change you can make in a person's self-esteem after you have enhanced their smile! People who love being orthodontists are generally gregarious and outgoing, but also enjoy focused critical thinking. Although we use instruments regularly, we are able to delegate significantly more clinical tasks to assistants than doctors in other specialties (or general dentistry), as the "heavy lifting" is mostly cerebral. Orthodontics requires a 2-3-year post-graduate residency program. Exact length depends on which program you attend.

Pediatric Dentistry: Obviously, this is the specialty that deals with diagnosis, treatment planning and dental treatment of children. First of all, primary (baby) teeth are different from permanent (adult) teeth in a number of ways. In addition, behavior management is a key differentiating factor between dealing with children as compared to adults. Pediatric dentists are highly knowledgeable and skilled at delivering treatment to children with diseases, syndromes and disabilities. These patients often require care to be rendered in a different manner, which may include sedation in a dental office or hospital. Pediatric dentists are usually fast-moving, upbeat, "bubbly" people who have a passion for caring for children, especially those who have special needs. Pediatric Dentistry requires a 2-year post-graduate residency program.

Periodontics: A periodontist is a specialist in all of the structures that support the teeth, including the gingiva (gums), alveolar bone (bone sockets that the teeth sit in) and the periodontal ligament (the structure that attaches the root of a tooth to the socket of bone that it is sitting in). Periodontists provide care and perform surgeries to improve the condition and/or orientation of the supporting structures. They are also highly skilled at placing bone grafts to fill voids in bone and implants to replace missing teeth. Periodontists are generally individuals who enjoy transforming an unhealthy mouth into one of stability. They are heavily involved the microbiology of the mouth, as much of what they correct is driven by the fact that an excess of harmful bacteria are doing damage to the patient's supporting structures. Periodontics requires a 3-year post-graduate residency program.

Endodontics: Endodontists are specialists in the structures found on the interior of teeth. Root canals make up the vast majority of the procedures they perform. The center of each tooth is where you find the pulp, which contains all the nerves and blood vessels found within a tooth. When the pulp becomes infected, a "root canal" must be done. During a root canal, the pulp is removed and replaced with a synthetic material. Endodontists have to be meticulous about what they do, as leaving any small amount of pulp generally results in a "flare-up," requiring another root canal to correct the error. Because it is difficult, often impossible to see all the way down to the bottom of the root of a tooth, endodontists depend largely on high-powered microscopes and x-rays to accomplish their tasks. Their work is very clinically technical, and they develop an extremely high level of dexterity as a result. Endodontists are intimately involved with microbiology, similarly to periodontists. They are usually highly detail-oriented people who enjoy taking on significant clinical challenges every day. They work in a quieter office environment and see less patients than most other specialists. Endodontics requires a 2-3-year post-graduate residency program. Exact length depends on which program you attend.

Prosthodontics: Prosthodontics is the specialty that deals with prosthetic devices used to replace missing teeth. The range of procedures a prosthodontist performs includes the process of designing and fabricating dentures and partial dentures, restoring implants (placing the fake tooth part of the implant into the mouth, adjusting it to fit just right with the other teeth and the bite, and securing it in place) and doing complex crown and bridge work. Prosthodontists often do large restorative cases where a patient needs lots of teeth replaced. In these cases, they must deal not only with all of the individual teeth that need restorations, but with how the bite will fit together when all the restorations are completed. This is extremely challenging and important, as great-looking teeth get you nowhere if they don't function properly. Prosthodontists spend large amounts of time doing lab work. Everything they do is completely custom and must be done to the finest level of detail. Prosthodontists are generally meticulous individuals who are willing do whatever is necessary to ensure their prostheses are of the highest quality. Prosthodontics requires a 3-year post-graduate residency program.

Oral and Maxillofacial Surgery: The specialty of oral surgery revolves around just that, surgery that is done in and around the mouth. Surgery can range from having a tooth pulled under local anesthesia (where the patient is given a shot to get numb, but not impaired/asleep), to orthognathic (jaw) surgery performed in a hospital setting under general anesthesia (where the patient is asleep), to removal of pathology like a cyst or tumor. Oral surgeons commonly extract third molars (wisdom teeth) and place implants. Since the range of procedures they can perform is vast, the training is the most extensive of any dental specialty. Oral surgery requires participation in either a 4-year or 6-year post-graduate training program. Graduates of the 6-year programs earn a Doctor of Medicine (M.D.) degree in addition to their dental doctorate degree (D.D.S or D.M.D.) they obtained when they completed dental school. In the 6-year programs, residents attend medical school for two years.

They take classes and tests with medical students, and I imagine it's a similar lifestyle to the first two years in dental school. The residents in 4-year programs do not go to medical school and thus do not graduate with an M.D. degree.

Dental Radiology: Dental Radiologists are specialists in the interpretation of radiographic images. This includes all different types of x-rays and MRIs, among others. Radiologists are well-versed not only in what structures are normal and which are abnormal in each type of radiograph, but also the benefits and shortfalls of each type of imaging. Dental radiologists generally never work in a traditional dental setting. Rather, they have a dark office with highly-sophisticated computer equipment, which allows them to receive images sent by general dentists or other specialists. They view the images under optimal conditions, analyze them, write a report of their findings and send it to the referring doctor. The referring doctor then reviews the radiologist's report and decides whether the condition in question requires intervention by herself, by another doctor, or does not require intervention at all. Dental radiology is unique in that the doctor rarely, if ever, puts on gloves or sees a patient in person. Dental Radiology requires a 2-year post-graduate residency program.

Dental Anesthesiology: Dental Anesthesiology is not recognized by the American Dental Association as a dental specialty. There are residencies offered after which doctors generally limit their practices specifically to dental anesthesia, however, so I believe this field should be described in this section. Just as with anesthesiology as a medical specialty, dental anesthesiologists have extensive knowledge and training in putting patients to sleep for dental procedures. A thorough knowledge of drugs used for this purpose and their reversal agents, how a patient is properly monitored when under general anesthesia, as well as how to respond in case of emergency are core tenets of a dental anesthesiologist. A doctor in this field works alongside another dentist for each procedure; he provides anesthesia to the patient while the dentist completes the necessary restorative work. It is common for him to work out of numerous offices, visiting each on its "anesthesia day," when it has all its patients scheduled who require anesthesia. Dental anesthesiologists put on gloves every day but never touch any dental instruments, as their work is completely limited to anesthesia. Dental Anesthesiology requires a 2-year post-graduate residency program.

I have extremely limited knowledge about the last two specialties, so I will use the American Dental Association's descriptions, as found on their website:

Oral Pathology: *Oral pathology is the specialty of dentistry and discipline of pathology that deals with the nature, identification, and management of diseases affecting the oral and maxillofacial regions. It is a science that investigates the causes, processes, and effects of these diseases. The practice of oral pathology includes research and diagnosis of diseases using clinical, radiographic, microscopic, biochemical, or other examinations.*

Dental Public Health: *Dental public health is the science and art of preventing and controlling dental diseases and promoting dental health through organized* *community efforts. It is that form of dental practice which serves the community as a patient rather than the individual. It is concerned with the dental health education of the public, with applied dental research, and with the administration of group dental care programs as well as the prevention and control of dental diseases on a community basis.*

Source: http://www.ada.org/en/education-careers/careers-in-dentistry/dental-specialties/specialty-definitions

Appendix B: D.D.S. vs. D.M.D., What's the Difference?

Nothing. The reason that they both exist is that for a long time, all dental school graduates earned their D.D.S. or Doctor of Dental Surgery degrees. Then, Harvard decided that they wanted to offer their dental graduates a different degree. I've heard it's because they didn't like how the Latin translation of Doctor of Dental Surgery sounded. I'm not sure if this is really true, but in any case, they came up with D.M.D., or Doctor of Dental Medicine. In English, this would abbreviate as D.D.M., but in Latin it's D.M.D., so they stick with that. As I said, there is no difference between the degrees, neither has an advantage over the other, and you shouldn't let the degree you'll receive have any influence on which dental school you attend.

Appendix C: Are Dentists Really Doctors?

Traditionally, when people use the term "doctor," they are referring to a medical doctor. The term "doctor" is also used to refer to a dentist, but for some, this comes with angst. In society, being a medical doctor is often thought of as reaching the apex of education, achievement and admiration. I've heard dentists referred to as "fake doctors," from time to time. I think this would make some of my colleagues pretty fired up, but I think it's kind of funny.

Here's my take on the situation: I don't like the fact that dentists go by "doctor" for several reasons: First of all, since everyone knows medical doctors as "doctors," it insinuates that dentists are trying to be the same. I've heard the opinion that dentists are individuals who could not get into medical school. I mean, maybe that's true for a few of us, but I think it is miles away from the truth for the vast majority. Dentistry and medicine are very different. Dentists utilize their hands and fine motor skills every day. Most medical doctors (surgeons excluded) do not. Dentists often own their own practices, and medical doctors generally work in large practices or hospitals. My belief of nearly all dentists, and I can say with confidence for myself, is that they *chose* to be dentists because they really wanted to do dentistry. I have all the respect in the world for medical doctors, as the work they do is 100% critical to preserve the health and well-being of people. What they do is amazing! It's just that being a medical doctor and being a dentist are two different jobs.

The way I see it, there are two sides to the term "doctor." The first, is that of respect; respect for the level of training and expertise a person has in his chosen field. For this reason, it is appropriate to call dentists "doctors." The other aspect of the term is one simply of reference to one's profession. Since medical doctors are generally referred to as "doctor," it makes it seem like dentists are trying to follow in their shadows (and in some people's eyes, falling short). I wish that way back when medical doctors were given the colloquial term "doctor," that dentists had been given the term "dentist" instead of "doctor." I know, I know, it would sound totally off the wall to refer to your dental practitioner as "Dentist Johnson," but if it had been this way from the get-go, it would sound normal and would carry the same level of respect that referring to your dentist as "Doctor Johnson" carries today. It is what it is though; the terminology is definitely not changing now. I just wanted to offer my take on the situation.

I don't see this issue as a big one, at all. I think only those with a serious need to be reminded of his accolades or, interpreted another way, someone with significant feelings of insecurity, would fixate on it. The take-home points are these: 1) Dentistry and medicine are two different fields and 2) The vast majority of people in each field *chose* to go into that field and were never relegated to it because they were unable to gain entry into the other field.

Appendix D: Useful Links and Contact Information

Useful Links:

American Dental Association (ADA):
https://www.ada.org/en

American Dental Education Association (ADEA): https://www.adea.org/

Applying to dental school:

- ADEA AADSAS Information and Application: https://www.adea.org/aadsas/
- Dental Admission Test (DAT) Information: https://www.ada.org/en/education-careers/dental-admission-test
- List of Dental Schools: https://www.asdanet.org/index/get-into-dental-school/before-you-apply/u-s-dental-schools

Financial Information:

- The White Coat Investor: https://www.whitecoatinvestor.com/
    - This is a website, blog, podcast, newsletter and book written by a practicing emergency physician who has gone to great lengths to educate himself in finance, particularly financial matters that pertain to high-earners like physicians and dentists. He offers numerous great, free resources (including

information about student loans!) to become educated in finance (HIGHLY recommended!).

- The Dough Roller Podcast with Rob Berger: https://www.doughroller.net/thepodcast/
    - This is a great introductory podcast to learn more about personal finance. Each podcast is focused on a specific topic, so it's easy to pick and choose where your time is best spent.

Contact Information:

I'm here to help and my offer does not end with the words in this book. If I can be of assistance to you in any way, please don't hesitate to reach out to me:

Leland Orthodontics

drleland@lelandorthodontics.com

(775) 900-9070

www.ingramcontent.com/pod-product-compliance
Lightning Source LLC
Chambersburg PA
CBHW022002170526
45157CB00003B/1107